NUTRIENT ADEQUACY

Assessment Using Food Consumption Surveys

Subcommittee on Criteria for Dietary Evaluation
Coordinating Committee on Evaluation of
Food Consumption Surveys
Food and Nutrition Board
Commission on Life Sciences
National Research Council

NATIONAL ACADEMY PRESS
Washington, D.C. 1986

NATIONAL ACADEMY PRESS ● 2101 Constitution Avenue, NW ● Washington, DC 20418

The work on which this publication is based was performed pursuant to Contract No. 59-3198-2-46 with the U.S. Department of Agriculture.

Library of Congress Catalog Card Number 85-62938

International Standard Book Number 0-309-03634-8

First Printing, December 1985
Second Printing, March 1987

Printed in the United States of America

Subcommittee on
Criteria for Dietary Evaluation

L. J. FILER, Jr. *(Chairman)*, University of Iowa College of Medicine, Iowa City, Iowa

GEORGE H. BEATON, Department of Nutritional Sciences, Faculty of Medicine, University of Toronto, Ontario, Canada

JACOB J. FELDMAN, National Center for Health Statistics, U.S. Department of Health and Human Services, Hyattsville, Maryland

HELEN A. GUTHRIE, Department of Nutrition, Pennsylvania State University, University Park, Pennsylvania

JEAN-PIERRE HABICHT, Division of Nutritional Sciences, Cornell University, Ithaca, New York

RICHARD HAVLIK, Clinical and Genetic Epidemiology Section, Division of Heart and Vascular Diseases, National Heart, Lung, and Blood Institute, National Institutes of Health, Bethesda, Maryland

D. MARK HEGSTED, Professor Emeritus, Harvard University, School of Public Health, Boston, Massachusetts

KENT K. STEWART, Department of Biochemistry and Nutrition, Virginia Polytechnic Institute and State University, Blacksburg, Virginia

HELEN SMICIKLAS-WRIGHT, Department of Nutrition, Pennsylvania State University, University Park, Pennsylvania

ANASTASIOS A. TSIATIS, Division of Biostatistics, Dana-Farber Cancer Institute, Boston, Massachusetts

National Research Council Staff

VIRGINIA HIGHT LAUKARAN, *Staff Officer,* Food and Nutrition Board

FRANCES M. PETER, *Editor,* Commission on Life Sciences

JUDITH GRUMSTRUP-SCOTT, *Editorial Consultant*

SUSHMA PALMER, *Executive Director*, Food and Nutrition Board

iii

Coordinating Committee on Evaluation of Food Consumption Surveys

Food and Nutrition Board

Preface

At the request of the U.S. Department of Agriculture (USDA), the National Research Council undertook a study of the criteria used to evaluate data on dietary intake. This study was performed by a subcommittee of the Coordinating Committee on Evaluation of Food Consumption Surveys. In January 1984, the subcommittee was formed to develop criteria for the use of survey data in the evaluation of dietary adequacy, paying particular attention to applications to data from the Nationwide Food Consumption Survey. During the course of its study, the subcommittee examined information on levels and variability of human nutrient requirements, survey methodology, and the reliability of food composition data.

Estimates of the proportion of the population with inadequate dietary intake have provided the impetus for food assistance programs and other efforts to improve the diet of the U.S. public. Increasingly, policymakers, scientists, and others interested in health maintenance recognize the need to improve the utilization of data on dietary intake and other information to monitor the U.S. population's nutritional status.

The proportion of the population at risk for inadequate nutrient intake can be estimated from survey data on dietary intake, even though the nutritional status of individuals can only be analyzed according to probabilities. The subcommittee in its deliberations developed an approach to dietary analysis that is based on these probabilities and takes into account the inherent variability of nutrient intake by individuals over time and of nutrients in the same foods.

Chapter 1 is a summary of the report. The history of dietary surveys is recounted in Chapter 2 along with a description of the committee's task and its approach to the study. In Chapter 3, the

vii

basis of dietary evaluation and its relationship to the recommended dietary allowances are discussed. The method of estimating usual dietary intake from survey data is described in Chapter 4. In Chapter 5, the recommended approach to dietary analysis is presented with examples. Chapter 6 deals with the application of the method in analysis of excessive intake and the utility of nutrient energy ratios. The impact of technical error on the analysis of dietary intake data is discussed in Chapter 7. Chapter 8 presents the results of confidence interval calculations. Chapter 9 is a summary of the subcommittee's recommendations. Additional details of the analyses described in the text are included in the appendices.

The committee gratefully acknowledges Susan Welsh, Betty Peterkin, and Robert L. Rizek of the USDA Human Nutrition Information Service (HNIS) for their interest and support; Brucy Gray, also of HNIS, for his preliminary analysis of the USDA data set; and Wayne Wolf and Joanne Holden of the Nutrient Composition Laboratory, USDA Beltsville Human Nutrition Center, for the reanalysis of their earlier work.

The subcommittee commends the able and dedicated assistance of the Food and Nutrition Board staff under the direction of Sushma Palmer, including staff officers Stephanie C. Crocco (prior to July 1984) and Virginia Hight Laukaran (beginning August 1984), and senior secretaries Sylvia Glasser and Tujuana M. Albritton. It is also grateful for the editorial assistance of Frances M. Peter and Judith Grumstrup-Scott.

L. J. FILER, JR.
Chairman
Subcommittee on Criteria
for Dietary Evaluation

Contents

xi

1
Executive Summary

Since 1936 the U.S. Department of Agriculture (USDA)
has been responsible for conducting periodic surveys of
food consumption. Currently, the agency's Nationwide
Food Consumption Survey (NFCS), a large study of the
food consumption patterns in the United States, includes
information on individual dietary intake, which serves
as a basis for determining the magnitude of inadequate
nutrition in the general population. To ensure that the
estimates of inadequacy are based on scientifically valid
parameters, the USDA asked the National Research Council
to develop criteria for the use of survey data in this
effort. As a result of this request, the Subcommittee on
Criteria for Dietary Evaluation was formed within the Food
and Nutrition Board of the Research Council's Commission
on Life Sciences.

The subcommittee was charged by the USDA with establishing criteria reflecting the degree of risk associated
with intakes of the following nutrients: ascorbic acid;
vitamins A, B_6, and B_{12}; calcium; folacin; iron; magnesium; riboflavin; niacin; phosphorus; thiamin; zinc; food
energy; and protein. The agency also requested that criteria be established for the evaluation of the proportion of
dietary intake derived from protein, fats, and carbohydrates as well as from total energy (caloric) intake. During the course of its study, the study group examined efforts
of the USDA and others in the scientific community to assess
the nutrient adequacy of diets in the U.S. population and
considered the analytic methods used in the past. Data from
the most recent NFCS survey were provided to the subcommittee to permit empirical testing of different approaches
for dietary evaluation.

USDA food assistance programs and other nutrition-related projects are based in part on estimates of inadequate nutrient intake derived from the NFCS. These estimates are also of interest to nutrition policymakers outside the USDA, scientists, and others who wish to identify population groups at risk of developing nutrient deficiency and to learn the determinants of unsatisfactory dietary intake for the country as a whole and for specific population groups. Although estimates based on dietary intake data are useful for examining adequacy of nutrient intake in a population or subpopulation, and may be useful in identifying individuals at relative risk of developing nutrient deficiency, they cannot be used alone to determine the nutritional status of individuals or population groups. For these purposes, biomedical and clinical measures are necessary.

The Recommended Dietary Allowances (RDAs) are often used as the basis for determining whether nutrient intake is adequate. They are standards for nutrient intake designed to meet the nutrient needs of virtually all healthy individuals in the United States. Because there is variation in nutrient needs among people despite similar physiological characteristics, margins of safety are built into the RDAs for many nutrients. Therefore, most people who receive less than the RDA for a specific nutrient will nevertheless meet their own nutrient requirement. For a number of years, a fixed cutoff point, such as two-thirds or three-fourths of the RDA, has been used by analysts to estimate the prevalence of inadequate intake for specific nutrients.

The subcommittee considered the merits of this type of analysis and concluded that it may lead to imprecise estimates, partly because it does not consider fully the variability in requirements among individuals. Consequently, some persons who are meeting their nutrient requirement may be judged by this method to have inadequate intake while some with inadequate intake will not be identified. A different approach based on the probability that a specific intake is inadequate to meet an individual's requirement was identified by the subcommittee, and guidelines were developed for interpreting the resulting estimates. Although the new approach is not difficult, it requires some familiarity with basic statistical theory. In this probability approach, estimates of average requirements and variability (i.e., the standard deviation) for the nutrient are used along with the shape of the distribution (e.g., normal or skewed) as the criteria for judging adequacy of dietary intake. The approach also requires information on the distribution of usual intakes among individuals examined in the survey. Dietary data from the NFCS are derived from interviews to determine the foods respondents have eaten for 3 days. Because the intake of an individual varies over time, it is necessary to adjust the distribution of dietary data in order to estimate the distribution of usual dietary intakes. The subcommittee also recognized that the analysis of nutrient intake adequacy may be constrained by systematic errors such as underreporting or overreporting of food intake and lack of information on the mean and shape of the requirement distribution for many nutrients.

The subcommittee believes that the prevalence of inadequate intake can be estimated for many nutrients and food components by using the probability approach. Empirical tests of the approach were made using intake data for iron, protein, vitamin A, and vitamin C in men and women and for thiamin in men. These data, from the 1977-1978 NFCS, were provided to the subcommittee by the USDA. The probability approach is not indicated for some nutrients, especially energy, as will be discussed below.

The overriding constraints in the application and interpretation of the probability approach are the limitations, validity, and reliability of estimates of mean nutrient requirements and survey data on dietary intake. At present, direct estimates of mean nutrient requirements are not available for most nutrients. Thus, the proposal to undertake probability analysis of dietary intake calls for the assignment of a higher priority to the development of the knowledge base on mean nutrient requirements and to improvement of the data on dietary intake by the collection of least two independent (i.e., nonconsecutive) observations for the same individuals. The subcommittee suggests that priority be assigned to the development of improved estimates of mean nutrient requirement for nutrients that a substantial proportion of the population is consuming at levels less than the RDA.

In the meantime, the subcommittee believes that the use of the probability approach will both stimulate and guide efforts to improve the validity and reliability of nutrient requirement estimates by permitting examination of the implications of different requirement estimates for a population, given current levels of dietary intake. There is now a need for further empirical testing of the proposed approach to determine the applicability of the method and to establish directions for further research.

MAJOR CONCLUSIONS

• The prevalence of inadequate intake can be estimated for many nutrients by the probability approach described in this report. For others, however, the method cannot be applied until research leads to a better understanding of both the average nutrient requirement and its variability, which are needed in probability analysis, and an improvement in the reliability of food composition data. These estimates are important in identifying determinants of inadequate intake, identifying possible interventions, and designing them for maximal efficiency. They are dependent on more comprehensive surveys to validate dietary analyses through biochemical and clinical measurements, such as are currently done in the National Health and Nutrition Examination Survey (NHANES) of the National Center for Health Statistics (NCHS).

• A basic statistical assumption of independence between requirement and intake is necessary for the probability approach. Thus, this method cannot be used meaningfully when the level of dietary intake and the required intake are correlated, as for dietary energy (calories), which most people in prosperous nations with low requirements consume at low levels. After reviewing the work of Lörstad (1971), however, the subcommittee concluded that this is not a problem.

• There is a need for continuing studies to improve research methods and thus data on dietary intake, which are essential for analysis regardless of the approach used. There is also a need for continuing attention to the validity of food composition data and research to improve such data.

• After examining the methods with which dietary intake data and reference data on the nutrient composition of foods are collected and conducting several types of analysis to determine the impact of random error, error due to the sampling technique, and systematic biases on the estimates of adequacy, the subcommittee concluded that such errors diminish the accuracy but do not necessarily destroy the utility of

estimates of the prevalence of inadequate intake. The
subcommittee believes that sensitivity testing is needed
to assist in determining which factors have the greatest
effect on prevalence estimates and hence should be given
priority for research to improve the approach.

MAJOR RECOMMENDATIONS

● Nutrient requirements based on multiple criteria of
adequacy should be developed and applied. For a given
nutrient, one might focus on the intake adequate to prevent clinical deficiency, to maintain functional integrity
of metabolic systems, and to maintain tissue stores. This
would permit multitiered population assessments.

If the probability approach is adopted, the following
suggestions should be considered when planning for future
NFCS surveys:

● Changes may be advisable in the design of food
intake data collection. For example, the number of 1-day
food intake observations per subject might be reduced; it
would be preferable to use the same data collection methods for each day of intake data; and it might be desirable
to avoid sampling on adjacent days and to continue to
sample on representative days of the week. These changes
should be made only after full consideration of all the
uses of the data and of the integration of survey planning
for all these purposes.

● Methods to reduce, or take into account, respondent
or interviewer bias should be developed to improve the
accuracy of food intake data.

● Continuing research on food intake methods and the
design of sampling strategies is recommended.

● Research should be conducted to determine the magnitude of any correlation between dietary intake and nutrient requirement.

● The subcommittee also recommends a number of actions
that should be considered in order to improve the reference
tables on nutrient composition of foods. These recommendations, which are presented in Chapter 9, relate to documen-
tation and analysis when data are missing, increases in sam-

ple size for nutrient composition analyses, and improvements in sampling methods.

● The design selected for future surveys should take into account all important uses of the survey data. The subcommittee's attention has been directed to one particular type of use. Other purposes may impose additional design demands on data collection approaches. The subcommittee believes that agencies responsible for the design and conduct of national or regional surveys would benefit from conducting analyses analogous to those discussed in this report, including full statistical consideration of the implication of design decisions on the precision and reliability of data analyses.

● It is imperative that future surveys include questions on intake of dietary supplements as well as of foods.

2

Introduction

Since 1936, the USDA has conducted six national surveys
of food consumption at roughly 10-year intervals. The
early surveys measured disappearance of food from household
supplies but not individual intake; however, in 1956 the
protocol was changed to include individual data on recall
of foods consumed over a 24-hour period. The latest
Nationwide Food Consumption Survey (NFCS), conducted in
1977-1978, included both household and individual components. It included a recall of foods consumed by individuals at home and away from home during a 3-day period.
The survey did not include questions on nutrient supplements. The data were collected through face-to-face
interviews during which individual household members were
asked to report their food intake over the previous 24
hours. The respondents were then given a food diary to
record their intake over the next 2 days. This individual
intake component consisting of a 1-day recall and 2-day
record for each individual is the basis for USDA analyses
of the nutritive value of foods consumed in the United
States (Peterkin et al., 1982). These data have been
reported by sex, age, region of residence, income, race,
and household characteristics (Pao et al., 1982).

For some years, the USDA used the recommended dietary
allowances (RDAs) (NRC, 1980) to evaluate the adequacy
of nutrient intake. However, the RDAs do not represent
the true requirement of all persons. Rather, they include a margin of safety to allow for variability and
other factors. Therefore, the USDA staff and other
food-consumption analysts have traditionally defined
inadequate intake as intake below a fixed cutoff point.
Some analysts use two-thirds of a specific RDA as a
definition of inadequate intake; others use one-half or

three-fourths of the RDA (Peterkin et al., 1982). There have been criticisms of this approach, and no clear rationale for the selection of the particular cutoff point has emerged.

Nutritional status cannot be determined from data on dietary intake alone. If appropriate criteria are used, however, these data can be used for making a preliminary evaluation of the proportion of the population that may be at risk for impaired nutritional status.

The task of the Subcommittee on Dietary Intake Evaluation was to develop criteria and approaches for interpreting the nutrient intake information in the Nationwide Food Consumption Survey (NFCS). Specifically, it was asked to develop criteria for using survey data on dietary intakes within the U.S. population or subpopulations in order to estimate the prevalence of inadequate nutrient intake. It did not examine methods to assess individual intakes or to determine the adequacy of an individual diet. In agreement with most analysts of survey data, the subcommittee determined that to assess dietary intake at the population level, it is necessary to compare the observed dietary intakes with the requirements for that nutrient.

The subcommittee began by examining previous efforts to estimate the prevalence of inadequate nutrient intake, focusing on the scientific merits of the approaches that have been taken. Recognizing that a probability approach had been used with apparent success for similar analytic problems (e.g., analysis of data on height and weight), the subcommittee tested the feasibility of this approach for analysis of dietary adequacy. During the course of its work, it became aware of the importance of three concepts for this kind of analysis:

● Because food and nutrient intakes vary from day to day, survey data on dietary intake must be adjusted to estimate statistically the distribution of usual dietary intake.

● Any approach to the assessment of dietary intake must take into account the mean and symmetry of the distribution of nutrient requirements among persons with similar characteristics. There is ample evidence that these nutrient requirements vary between persons in

similar categories of age, sex, body weight, and pregnancy
and lactation status.

● Because changes in physiological or functional
criteria for nutrient requirements require changes in the
level of dietary intake needed to meet the requirement,
any approach to interpreting intake in relation to requirement must incorporate a definition of the criterion the
requirements are intended to satisfy. It is possible, and
indeed desirable, to define multiple criteria of adequacy,
multiple levels of requirement, and hence a multitiered
population assessment.

Chapters 3 and 4 of this report address these issues
and are followed in Chapter 5 by a discussion of the
proposed analytic method, including examples of applications to selected nutrients. The subcommittee also
recognized other important uses for data on food consumption, including the identification of food patterns associated with inadequate dietary intake and the determination of changes in eating patterns that are likely to be
acceptable, feasible, and economical for groups with poor
diets. This kind of information is needed to design food
assistance programs and meal patterns for these programs,
to encourage improvements in nutrition education, and to
design nutrition intervention programs mandated by law.
Information on food consumption patterns is also essential
for the development of food safety regulations, which are
promulgated by the Food and Drug Administration (FDA) and
the Environmental Protection Agency (EPA). These uses,
although not germane to this report, are as important as
estimating the prevalence of inadequate intake and are a
major function of the NFCS and other dietary intake surveys. The subcommittee has cautioned that the final design
of future surveys must take into account all the intended
uses of the data--not just assessment of the prevalence of
inadequate intakes discussed in this report.

3

Nutrient Requirements as a Basis for Dietary Evaluation

When using nutrient requirements as a basis for dietary evaluation, a number of factors must be considered. For example, there is great variability among similar people as well as different interpretations of adequacy and deficiency. All these factors must be considered in order to use nutrient requirements most effectively.

VARIABILITY OF NUTRIENT REQUIREMENTS

Like all other biological features, nutrient requirements vary among seemingly similar persons. Although variability generally applies to all nutrients, its nature is known to be specific to certain nutrients.

Dietary standards are usually described as recommended dietary allowances, safe levels of intake, or other similar terms. A distinction must be made between these and the term requirements, which is used in this report. Over the past few decades, groups charged with the development of standards for dietary intake recognized the variability of nutrient requirements; nevertheless, they designated a single point in the distribution as the recommended dietary allowance (RDA) (FAO/WHO/UNU, in press; Health and Welfare, Canada, 1983; NRC, 1980). For protein, for example, a single point was chosen to estimate the dietary intake level adequate to meet the needs of almost all healthy persons in a specified age or sex group. The point was established after examining the data base for each nutrient and then making scientific judgments about the position and nature of the requirement distribution. By definition, the point chosen to meet the needs of almost all persons lies near the upper tail of the requirement distribution (NRC, 1974).

When there is information on which to base inferences about the actual distribution, as for protein, the mean plus 2 SD has been identified as the recommended intake (FAO/WHO/UNU, in press; Health and Welfare, Canada, 1983; NRC, 1980). For most nutrients, the distribution has not been explicitly described, and the relationship between recommended intake and requirement distribution has not been explored in detail. The principle still holds, however, that the recommended intake level generally exceeds the estimated requirements and, hence, the needs of almost all persons.

Dietary standards for energy intake are different from those for specific nutrients because the level published for energy is usually the estimated mean requirement, i.e., one-half of the persons are expected to have higher needs and one-half, lower needs (FAO/WHO/UNU, in press; Health and Welfare, Canada, 1983). Some reports provide a range around the median energy requirement (NRC, 1980); others present an estimate of the variance of energy requirements (FAO/WHO/UNU, in press; Health and Welfare, Canada, 1983).

Nutrient requirements of specific persons can only be expressed by referring to the probability (FAO/WHO/UNU, in press) or likelihood that each level of observed intake is inadequate. In a probability approach, therefore, the underlying distribution of requirements among similar persons must be recognized. This is in contrast to using a fixed cutoff point delineating inadequate from adequate nutrient intake, which fails to recognize those persons whose intake and requirement may both be below the cutoff point. If the cutoff point is set below the RDA, both intake and requirement of some persons may be higher than the cutoff point.

The period during which a specified requirement must be met is seldom defined (FAO/WHO/UNU, in press; Health and Welfare, Canada, 1983). Requirement estimates are usually related more generally to levels of usual or habitual intake (FAO/WHO/UNU, in press; Health and Welfare, Canada, 1983; NRC, 1980). They do not refer to intake on a particular day, unless that is a reliable measure of the usual intake. Nutrient requirements as used for the analysis in this report consist of a distribution of usual dietary intakes required to maintain an adequate or acceptable physiological or nutritional state.

For a few nutrients, requirement information simply is not available, and meaningful analysis of the adequacy of dietary intake must await the development of further knowledge of requirement distributions. For others, there is some information, but its precision may be low. Nevertheless, coupling available information about requirement with other information about factors expected to affect requirement can permit the development of informed judgments about requirements for various age and sex groups. As a result, it should be feasible to use a probability approach to improve present inferences about the adequacy of dietary intake. It is important that priority be given to the nutrients that are most likely to present public policy problems in the United States.

For a few nutrients and age groups, better information about requirements appears to be available, and one can be more confident in their application. On the whole, however, there is a clear need for research on nutrient requirements. It is important that priority be given to those nutrients which are most likely to present public policy problems in the United States. Such refinement should permit the development of improved statistical approaches to survey interpretation through the use of information about nutrient requirements. Until exact information about requirements is available, the resultant inferences about prevalence must be considered imprecise, although the probability approach is superior to other possible methods.

Information about mean requirements and characteristics of their distributions for some but not all nutrients may be found in the reports of committees charged with developing recommended intakes. However, the development and presentation of information needed for all nutrients have not been included in the mandate to such committees. This does not mean that the information is unavailable but, rather, that it may be necessary to undertake a special effort to examine the literature and develop the required data base. The present subcommittee did not attempt such a search and notes that skills and experience not represented in its membership would be needed to perform the requisite task.

LEVELS OF REQUIREMENT

Multiple definitions of adequacy are possible (e.g., the prevention of clinical deficiency symptoms, the main-

tenance of specified levels of the nutrients or their
metabolites in tissues, the maintenance of enzyme activity
at specified levels), and each of these could be associated with a different dietary requirement. Thus, it is
possible to establish a family of requirement curves
marking different definitions of adequacy.

Estimates of average requirement based on these different criteria can be derived from the early nutrition
literature. The earliest marker for nutritional adequacy
was the prevention of clinically detectable signs of malfunction. Estimates based on deficiency avoidance were
provided in some early dietary standards, along with
recommended intakes for improved nutrition, e.g., in the
1963 Dietary Standard for Canada (Committee on Revision of
the Canadian Dietary Standard, 1964). Recent RDA reports
(NRC, 1980) provide some of the information needed for the
proposed approach. Such information can also be found in
reports issued by FAO and WHO (e.g., FAO/WHO, 1967, 1970).

Throughout the world, dietary standards and recommended
intakes are based on basic philosophies that differ in
detail (IUNS, 1983a,b) but have a similar goal of establishing levels of intake that will maintain a state of
nutriture beyond the mere prevention of clinical deficiency
disease. For example, adequate iron intakes are regarded
as those that maintain reasonable iron stores rather than
those that merely stabilize mild anemia or maintain hemoglobin at physiologically normal levels (FAO/WHO, 1970;
Health and Welfare Canada, 1983; NRC, 1980). Similarly,
vitamin C requirements have been set at a level that is
sufficient to establish and maintain metabolic pools
(Health and Welfare Canada, 1983; NRC, 1980) or to maintain tissue levels (FAO/WHO, 1970) rather than just to
prevent scurvy. Requirements for other nutrients are
determined in analogous ways. The criteria selected for
the same nutrient often vary between reports, even within
the same country (e.g., ascorbic acid in Canada).

Levels of intake and requirement estimates lower than
those given in many recently published dietary standards
appear to be consistent with the absence of clinical signs
of ill health. Thus, some definitions of requirement may
be more desirable that others, depending on the purposes
of the dietary assessment. Interpretations of dietary
intake data in relation to estimated requirements require
consideration of the particular biochemical, physical,

clinical, or functional criteria that were used to establish the requirement.

A multilevel assessment procedure can be used by developing a series of requirement distribution estimates, each referring to a defined criterion of adequacy. By using the several requirements, one can calculate a series of estimates of the prevalence of inadequate intakes. Although the RDA reports may not provide the appropriate information for determining such a family of requirement estimates, this absence does not mean that the information is not available. Such information may not have been presented because those reports are intended primarily for use in developing a single requirement to meet the needs of all healthy individuals.

FIXED CUTOFF POINTS

It is a common practice to use fixed cutoff points to estimate the adequacy of nutrient intake. In this method, estimates of the prevalence of inadequate intake have been based on a fixed proportion of the RDA. The rationale has been based on the recognition that the RDAs, designed to include virtually all healthy individuals, have included margins of safety--often generous margins. Hence, if applied as a criterion, an RDA would clearly lead to an overestimate of the prevalence of inadequacy. Therefore, the proportions selected as cutoffs have varied--sometimes two-thirds, sometimes three-quarters, and sometimes 70%. There has not been a clear rationale for the selection of the level.

The use of fixed cutoff points is conceptually similar to population-based screening for unrecognized disease (e.g., Rogan and Gladen, 1978). The well-known terms used to describe problems of medical screening are similar to those encountered with the use of cutoff points (Habicht, 1980). Thus, both the terms and the screening approach have been used to examine the fixed cutoff point method.

Regardless of the cutoff point selected, some persons who meet their nutrient requirement will be identified as having inadequate intake. Conversely, some who do not meet their requirement will be identified as adequately nourished. The term sensitivity is applied to the ability of a test to detect truly affected individuals; specifi-

<u>city</u> refers to the ability of a test to identify truly
unaffected individuals. Misclassification occurs when
people are designated <u>not</u> <u>at</u> <u>risk</u> when they are truly
affected by the condition (false negatives) or <u>at</u> <u>risk</u>
when they are actually unaffected (false positives). In
statistical decision-making, a similar concept is used,
with sensitivity and specificity corresponding to Type I
(α) and Type II (β) errors in hypothesis testing. In
Figure 3-1, the distribution of those who truly fail to
meet their requirement and the distribution of those who
truly meet their requirement are plotted. For the purpose
of illustration, it is assumed that persons can be classified with an absolutely accurate test.

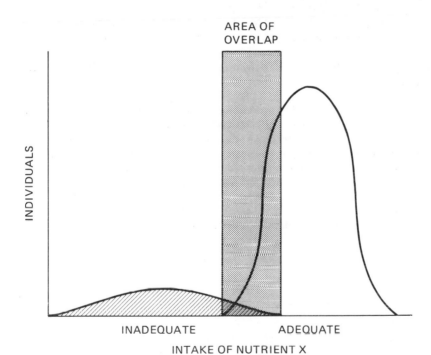

FIGURE 3-1. The distributions of people who truly fail
to meet their requirement (inadequate) and
those who truly meet it (adequate) for a
hypothetical nutrient X.

This figure is useful in gaining an understanding of the implications of the fixed cutoff point approach. Presumably, a cutoff point would be selected somewhere in the area of overlap between the distribution of truly adequate and truly inadequate intake. For this to be done, the sensitivity and specificity of the cutoff point would have to be determined (Habicht et al., 1982). Brownie and Habicht (1984) have developed a strategy for selecting the optimal cutoff point under certain conditions.

The most important conclusion from these considerations (Brownie and Habicht, 1984) is that the choice of the optimal cutoff point to estimate prevalence or changes in prevalence depends upon a rather exact estimate of the prevalence being sought--an impossibility. Estimates of prevalence using less than optimal cutoff points can be corrected (Rogan and Gladen, 1978) by taking the sensitivity and specificity of the cutoff point into account. Although this approach is theoretically possible, no such data are presently available and, more importantly, it is probably impracticable to acquire such data with the precision required. It is not rational to select the cutoff as a proportion of the highest requirement in the population.

When fixed cutoff points are used without these corrections, estimation of the prevalence of inadequate intake is in error and the magnitude, the extent, and even the direction of the error cannot be estimated. Recognizing the drawbacks in the use of fixed cutoff points, the subcommittee concluded that a different approach was required to analyze the adequacy of dietary intake. The probability approach proposed in this report avoids the limitations of the fixed cutoff points.

4

The Use of Short-Term Dietary Intake Data to Estimate Usual Dietary Intake

Dietary intake of an individual is not constant from day to day but varies both in amount and in type of foods eaten and, hence, in nutrient content (intraindividual variation). There are also variations between persons in their usual nutrient intake averaged over time (interindividual variation). For North American populations, the intraindividual variation is usually as large as or greater than interindividual variations and must be taken into account in any approach to nutrient assessment.

RELATIONSHIP OF DAILY DIETARY INTAKE DATA TO USUAL INTAKE

Many authors have compared the reliability of data from 1-day dietary intake records and records for longer periods (Garn et al., 1978; Marr, 1971; Pekkarinen, 1970; Young et al., 1952a), and errors in usual intake estimation due to intraindividual variation have attracted considerable interest. Initially, the interest of scientists was stimulated by the desire to examine biological relationships in epidemiological data sets, for example, dietary intake and serum lipid levels or energy intake and lipid levels (Beaton, 1982a; Beaton et al., 1979; Jacobs et al., 1979; Liu et al., 1978; Stallones, 1982). At about the same time, several researchers realized that when 1-day dietary intake data are used, intraindividual intake variation results in a serious bias in regression and correlation analyses. This bias can easily lead to false conclusions about the underlying biological relationships (Beaton, 1982b; Beaton et al., 1979; Jacobs et al., 1979; Liu et al., 1978; Sempos et al., 1985; Stallones, 1982). The concept of measurement error and the statistical approaches for dealing with it are not new. It has been applied in other fields for many

17

years. However, there is new appreciation of the applicability of these concepts to data on dietary intake.

As a result of the phenomenon of intraindividual variation, when one uses a fixed cutoff point for an observed intake distribution, the number of days on which intake was recorded affects the apparent prevalence of inadequate intake (Hegsted, 1972). Figure 4-1 illustrates the impact of repeated observations on the apparent distribution of intakes and on the apparent prevalence of intakes falling below a fixed cutoff point.

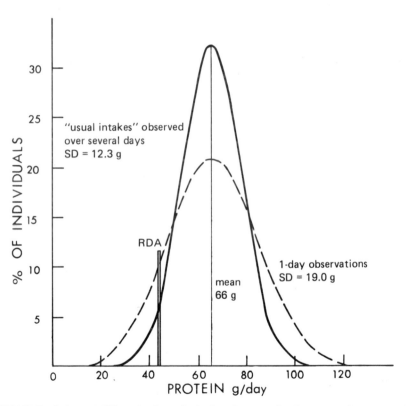

FIGURE 4-1. Effect of multiple days of observation on the apparent distribution of nutrient intake. From Hegsted, 1972. Reprinted by permission of the author and publishers. Copyright © Gordon and Breach Science Publishers, Inc.

Interest in the magnitude of this day-to-day variation in intake continued in recent years (Beaton et al., 1979, 1983; Hackett et al., 1983; Houser and Bebb, 1981; Hunt et al., 1983; Karvetti and Knuts, 1981; Liu et al., 1978; McGee et al., 1982; Rush and Kristal, 1982; Sempos et al., 1985; Todd et al., 1983). Earlier reports addressed the same issue with specific reference to estimating energy intake or ways to derive information about energy and lipid components (Balogh et al., 1971; Hankin et al., 1967; Kato et al., 1973; Keys, 1970; Marr, 1971; Morris et al., 1963; Tillotson et al., 1973). These reports indicate that the magnitude of the intraindividual component, relative to the interindividual component, varies with nutrient; probably with the age, sex, and sociocultural group; and with dietary methodology. This is illustrated in Table 4-1, which presents the ratio of intra- to interindividual variance for various studies by nutrient and sex. Several authors noted that for nutrients with markedly skewed distributions, the ratios for logarithmically transformed intake distributions were lowered (Beaton et al., 1983; Hunt et al., 1983; Sempos et al., 1985). The table shows a consistency in the ratio of intra- to interindividual variation, in that most nutrients for all five studies produced values greater than 1. However, the data of Hackett et al. (1983) for a group of children suggest generally higher ratios for energy, protein, total fat, and total carbohydrate. In addition, there seems to be some difference between males and females and between various nutrients. The method of assessing dietary intake may have affected the ratio of the variances, since true random error would be included in the intraindividual component.

In a recent study by Sempos et al. (1985), dietary data were collected for a sample of 15 women who completed two randomly selected 1-day records per month for a total of 29 records during a period of 2 years. The data were then analyzed for each year (Table 4-1). The various ratios were very similar in each year, suggesting that there were stable characteristics within the population. These authors demonstrated that the variance ratio does reflect the true usual intake and day-to-day variation and validates other studies of shorter duration.

Both Hunt et al. (1983) and Sempos et al. (1985) noted that use of nutrient supplements altered the variance ratios. Sempos et al. (1985) found ratios less than 1 and usually less than 0.5 for iron, thiamin, riboflavin, niacin,

TABLE 4-1. Observed Ratios[a] of Intraindividual and Interindividual Variances[b]

Nutrient	24-Hour Recall by Young Adults[c]	3-Day Record by Older Adults[d]	1-Day Recall by Women[e] Year 1	1-Day Recall by Women[e] Year 2	7-Day Record by Men[f]	24-Hour Recall by Pregnant Women[g]
Males:						
Energy	1.1	1.0			0.8	
Protein	1.5	1.2			1.4	
Carbohydrate	1.6	2.1			0.6	
Fat	1.2	1.2			1.3	
SFA[h]	1.1	2.2			1.4	
PUFA[i]	2.8	3.5			1.9	
Cholesterol	3.4	5.6			1.6	
Vitamin A	[j]	1.6				
Vitamin C	3.5	2.3				
Thiamin	2.5	0.9				
Riboflavin	2.4	0.9				
Niacin	1.6	2.2				
Calcium	2.2	1.1				
Iron	1.7	1.8				
Females:						
Energy	1.4	0.8	1.6	1.6		1.1
Protein	1.5	1.3	2.1	2.1		1.4
Carbohydrate	1.4	1.2	NR[k]	NR		1.2
Fat	1.6	0.9	NR	NR		1.2
SFA[h]	1.4	1.7	NR	NR		NR
PUFA[i]	4.0	2.2	NR	NR		NR
Cholesterol	4.3	4.2	NR	NR		NR
Vitamin A	24.3	2.5	7.7	10.9		NR
Vitamin C	2.0	2.8	2.3	2.5		NR
Thiamin	4.4	1.6	3.3	3.9		NR
Riboflavin	2.2	1.8	3.0	3.3		NR
Niacin equivalent	4.0	2.5	NR	NR		NR
Calcium	0.9	1.7	1.1	1.2		1.0
Iron	2.5	1.5	2.7	2.5		NR

[a]A ratio of 1.0 indicates that the intraindividual and interindividual variances are equal. A ratio greater than one indicates that intraindividual variance is greater than interindividual variance.
[b]The original papers contain additional data. Only those nutrient variables examined in two or more papers are included here.
[c]From Beaton et al., 1979, 1983.
[d]From Hunt et al., 1983.
[e]From Sempos et al., 1985.
[f]From McGee et al., 1982.
[g]From Rush et al., 1982.
[h]Saturated fatty acids.
[i]Polyunsaturated fatty acids.
[j]None of the variance could be assigned to subjects.
[k]NR=Not reported.

and vitamin C (as well as for some other nutrients not included in Table 4-1) when food intakes with supplements were analyzed.

PROCEDURE FOR ADJUSTING INTAKE DATA

When the intraindividual variation of dietary intake and the number of days of observation are known, it is possible to determine reliability of dietary intake data for each particular person. The usual intake for each person lies within the bounds described by the following equation 95% of the time if the day-to-day variations are normally distributed:

$$\pm 2 \times SD \text{ (intra)}/ \sqrt{n},$$

where SD (intra) is the measure of intraindividual variation and n is the number of observations for the individual person. The following discussion assumes normally distributed (Gaussian) data, even though this is rarely the case with food intake data. The appropriate transformations to obtain Gaussian distributions are discussed later.

When the number of days of observation increases from 1 to 4, the confidence limits are reduced by one-half, and the reliability of the estimate of usual dietary intake is improved accordingly. If one considers the actual magnitude of intraindividual variation, however, the results are somewhat disheartening. For example, the intraindividual coefficient of variation for energy in adults is approximately 25% of the mean (Beaton et al., 1979). This suggests that about 3 weeks of intake data are needed to estimate usual energy intake with confidence limits of approximately ±10%.

When determining usual intakes in populations, there is a need not for reliable estimates of the dietary intake for each person but, rather, for reliable estimates of the distribution of usual intakes for the population (Hegsted, 1972). Unlike individual intakes, the distribution of usual dietary intakes for the population can be approximated from a modest number of repetitions of the 1-day intake data; however, seasonal variations in intake and variation between weekdays and weekend days must also be taken into account in the data collection.

The overall variability in a distribution of dietary intake can be described in the following terms:

$$V(total) = V(inter) + V(intra)/n,$$

where V(total) = total variance of data (square of observed SD), V(inter) = between-subject variance, V(intra) = within-subject variance or residual error term in an analysis of variance, and n = number of days of intake data. In this equation, the interindividual variation represents the distribution of usual intake referred to previously.

Statistical theory allows us to derive an estimate of the distribution of usual intakes, given the observed mean, the total variance, and an estimate of the intraindividual variance. Replicated observations of 1-day dietary intake are needed to obtain an estimate of intraindividual variation. In theory, the replicated observations should be independent of one another in time rather than on consecutive days, although it is not yet known whether this is important in practice.

The magnitude of the intraindividual variation can be estimated by analysis of variance (ANOVA). If the original distribution is not normal, the distribution must be transformed into a more normal form before the ANOVA procedure is applied. (See Appendix A for an example of a logarithmic transformation for this purpose.) To adjust the intake distribution, the deviation of each point from the population mean is multiplied by the ratio of the interindividual standard deviation to observed standard deviation. With this nonparametric procedure, it is not necessary to assume a perfect fit of the normal distribution, and the distinctive shape of the original distribution is preserved. The adjusted data are then transformed back to the original scale for subsequent analyses. Figures 4-2 and 4-3 depict two distributions derived from Nationwide Food Consumption Survey (NFCS) data that have been adjusted to estimate the distribution of usual dietary intake of protein for males and iron for females.

Appendix A provides full details of the approach used in generating distributions for this report. Although ANOVA is not recommended as the only approach to estimating interindividual variation and eliminating the effects of day-to-day variability, it can serve as an example of possible

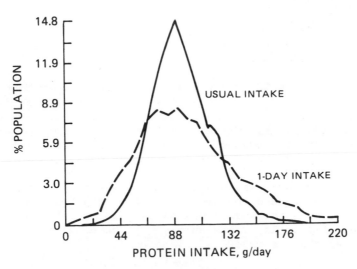

FIGURE 4-2. Comparison of 1-day and adjusted distributions
for protein intake by male adults. Derived
from the 1977-1978 NFCS data analysis described
in Appendix A.

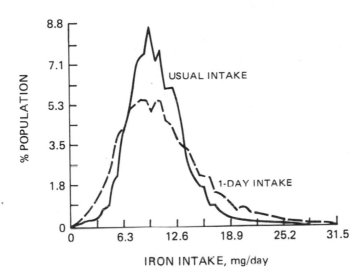

FIGURE 4-3. Comparison of 1-day and adjusted distributions
for iron intake by female adults. Derived from
the 1977-1978 NFCS data analysis described in
Appendix A.

approaches (Trumpler and Weaver, 1953). The method of normalizing the original distribution should be appropriate to the data set under study (Box and Cox, 1964).

The current NFCS is designed to collect information for 3 consecutive days for all subjects. There is a possibility that dietary intake on consecutive days is correlated within the individual. If this is true, the statistical power of the estimates is reduced. On the other hand, the subcommittee believes that 3 days of observation may be more than is required for the derivation of the distribution of usual intakes. For purposes other than the analysis of dietary adequacy, such as using dietary intake data for multivariate analysis, data for additional days would probably be required. All goals of the survey must be considered when the final decision is made.

In summary, the impact of day-to-day variation in intake contributes to errors in estimations of usual intake. If the survey data include an adequate number of independent replicate observations of intake measurements, methods can be used to adjust the observed intake distribution to generate a good estimate of the distribution of usual intakes. In a large survey, such as the NFCS, this approach is feasible and may even permit collection of fewer data than are now collected, given an appropriate sampling design. The feasibility of this reduction depends, of course, on other uses of the data. For example, if providing descriptive data on patterns of food use other than intake is a purpose of the survey, more replications may be needed. There is no need to collect more days of dietary data per individual than in the recent NFCS to implement the analytical approach described in this chapter for adjustment of the intake distributions. The only additional cost involves the statistical resources needed to design and analyze the data.

5

The Probability Approach

Recognizing the weaknesses of previous efforts to analyze dietary intake, the subcommittee sought an approach
that would take into account the variability both in usual
nutrient intake among individuals and in their nutrient
requirements. To meet this need, it developed and eval-
uated a probability approach based on a comparison of two
distributions: nutrient requirement and nutrient intake.
This method takes into account the likelihood that persons
with a particular level of intake would fail to meet their
nutrient requirement. The probability of inadequate intake
would naturally be very low for those with higher nutrient
intakes and would be higher for those with lower nutrient
intake.

Figure 5-1 shows the distribution of protein requirements among adult men. The probability curve for the intake has been plotted as a cumulative distribution of
requirement. At the lower level of intake, below the lower
tail of the original distribution, intake should be inadequate to meet requirements for everyone. (No persons are
believed to have requirements that low.) At the level of
the mean requirement, assuming a symmetrical distribution,
half the individuals would be expected to have higher needs
and half lower. In the upper tail of the distribution,
probability of inadequacy approaches zero. (No persons are
believed to have requirements this high.) From Figure 5-1,
then, a probability of inadequacy can be assigned to any
observed level of usual intake. The probability or risk
curve is specific to a particular class of people--in this
figure, adult men. The application of this concept to
protein is discussed in detail in the FAO/WHO/UNU (in
press) report on energy and protein requirements.

25

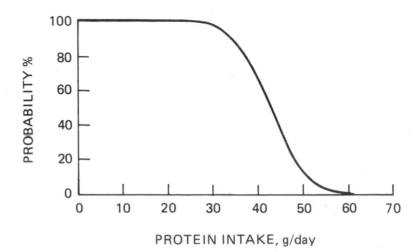

FIGURE 5-1.   Cumulative distribution of protein requirement
expressed as a probability curve. The curve
describes the probability, or risk, that an
observed intake would be inadequate for a randomly selected male, assuming a normal distribution of protein requirements.   Based on NRC,
1980.

In Figure 5-1, the probability of inadequate intake is
plotted against the protein intake for an adult male.
Beyond approximately 30 g/day, the probability of inadequate intake decreases rapidly and reaches zero at an
intake of about 60 g/day. When applied to the distribution of intakes observed in a population, the curve can
be used to generate a prediction or estimate of the prevalence of inadequate intakes. The approach does not identify those particular individuals who have inadequate
intakes, only the proportion of the population.

When the approach was applied to iron, Beaton (1974)
demonstrated that predictions of the prevalence of inadequate iron intakes seemed consistent with estimates based
on hematologic data on the proportion of women who might
be expected to have increased hemoglobin levels when
treated with iron. In that analysis, approximately 75% of
women in the sample had intakes less than the Canadian
recommended intake of 14 mg/day, but only about 15% were
predicted to have intakes below their own requirements
(Beaton 1971, 1974). The approach for iron is discussed

in Appendix B and is used with data from the Nationwide Food Consumption Survey (NFCS) later in this section.

More recently, the joint FAO/WHO/UNU (in press) committee that studied protein requirements accepted the principles of the probability approach and suggested that it be applied to the interpretation of observed protein intakes. That committee emphasized that the approach cannot easily be applied to energy. In essence, any logistically simple approach depends on the assumption that the correlation between intake and requirement is approximately known among similar individuals. On the basis of existing data, this is a reasonable assumption for the nutrients, at least after body weight or other common denominator variables of requirement are taken into account. There is no a priori reason to believe that the person with a low (or high) usual intake will necessarily have a low (or high) requirement. It is possible then to assign a probability of inadequacy to observed intake of nutrients. However, much evidence suggests that usual energy intake and expenditure are closely related in most people (Beaton, 1983; FAO/WHO/UNU, in press). That is, a person with a low energy intake is very likely the person with low energy expenditure. One would have to know the magnitude of this substantial correlation before a probability approach could be applied to energy with any degree of confidence. Obtaining this information would be very difficult in the general population.

A specific example of the probability approach applied to protein intake is presented in Table 5-1. The adjusted distribution of protein intakes using 1977-1978 NFCS data provided to the subcommittee (Figure 4-2) has been arbitrarily divided into 11 intake intervals. For each intake interval, the percentage of the total population expected to have inadequate intakes is estimated by multiplying the percentage of the total population in that intake interval (frequency distribution) by the probability of inadequate intake for that interval. When the percentages of inadequate intake at each level are added together, the sum is 2.2%--the estimated prevalence of inadequate protein intakes for that population of adult males (Table 5-1).

The probabilities portrayed in Figure 5-1 and tabulated in Table 5-1 were derived from the description of protein requirements provided in the Recommended Dietary Allowances (NRC, 1980). The average protein requirements were stipu-

TABLE 5-1. Predicted Proportion of Adult Males with
Protein Intakes Below Their Individual
Requirements: An Application of the Proba-
bility Approach[a]

Intake Interval (and Midpoint), g/day	Percentage of Total Population with Observed Intake in That Interval[b]	Z Value[c]	Probability of Inadequacy[d]	Estimated Percentage of Total Population with Inadequate Intake[e]
24	0.4	−2.85	1.0	0.4
24–28 (26)	0.1	−2.53	0.995	0.1
28–32 (30)	0.2	−1.90	0.97	0.19
32–36 (34)	0.2	−1.27	0.90	0.18
36–40 (38)	0.5	−0.63	0.74	0.37
40–44 (42)	0.9	0	0.5	0.45
44–48 (46)	1.1	+0.63	0.26	0.29
48–52 (50)	1.3	+1.27	0.10	0.13
52–56 (54)	1.8	+1.90	0.03	0.05
56–60 (58)	3.5	+2.53	0.005	0.02
60	91.0[f]	+2.86	0	0
			Total	2.2[g]

[a]Based on 1977–1978 NFCS data provided to the subcommittee.
[b]Based on frequency distribution.
[c]Z value = interval midpoint − mean requirement/SD.
[d]Probabilities for each Z value; determined by identifying area to right of Z in tables of standard normal distribution.
[e]Obtained by multiplying probability of inadequacy by
proportion of population in each interval.
[f]Percentages do not add to 100 due to rounding.
[g]Prevalence of inadequate protein intake in this population of adult males. Obtained by adding the percentages for each interval.

lated as 0.6 g/kg body weight/day with a coefficient of
variation (CV) of 15%. When this was applied to a 70-kg
man in the RDA report, the mean requirement was 42 g/day
and the SD, 6.3 g/day. Using these parameters and a table
of areas under the normal distribution curve, one can
derive the proportion of individuals with actual requirement above a specified level of intake, X. These values

are portrayed in Figure 5-1. This approach was applied to population data by Anderson et al. (1984).

The sample analysis in Table 5-1 is based on relatively wide ranges of intake. Through the use of computers, very narrow intervals can be analyzed, thus improving the accuracy of the estimates. Only 11 intervals were used in Table 5-1 because of the constraints of space in this report. The use of such a small number of intake levels is not recommended but is unlikely to cause major error. In its other analyses, the subcommittee analyzed 200 intake intervals. If a parametric approach is used, the actual distributions rather than points on the distribution are analyzed. This approach is examined in Chapter 8 and Appendix C.

The approach can be used with any known distribution function. For example, the distribution of menstrual iron losses is a major determinant of iron requirement in females. This distribution approximates the log-normal distribution. By logarithmic transformations of the data on iron intake and use of the logarithmic requirement distribution, a probability approach analogous to the one described above can be applied. Figure 5-2 portrays the probability, or risk, curve for inadequate iron intake by menstruating women, derived as described in Appendix B.

REQUIREMENT INFORMATION NEEDED FOR THE PROBABILITY APPROACH

A knowledge of, or a reasonable assumption about, the mean and shape of the requirement distribution for a particular nutrient is necessary for the probability approach to be applied. As discussed above, the underlying assumption of the method is that the correlation between nutrient intake and requirement is low within reasonably homogeneous groups of people. Where this is not true, as for energy, the strength of the correlation must be estimated.

For many nutrients, precise descriptions of mean requirement are not available. Indeed, presumably reliable descriptions are available only for protein and vitamin A in adults (NRC, 1980) and for iron in menstruating women (FAO/WHO, 1970; Health and Welfare, Canada, 1983). For other age and physiological groups and for other nutrients, there may be reasonable estimates of the mean requirement, the range of requirements, or perhaps both, but little or no direct knowl-

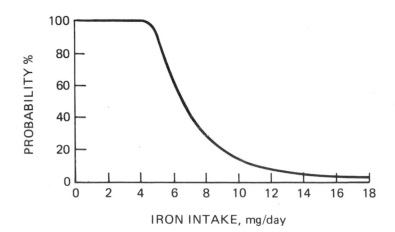

FIGURE 5-2. Probability curve for iron intake in menstruating females. The curve describes the
probability, or risk, that an observed level
of iron intake would be inadequate to meet
the needs of a randomly selected female.
This curve is based on the assumption that
that menstrual loss follows a log-normal
distribution. Based on 1977-1978 NFCS data
provided to the subcommittee. (Analysis
discussed in Appendix B.)

edge about the shape of the requirement distribution. In
this situation, it is instructive to determine through
sensitivity analysis the effect of a particular assumption
on the outcome of the analysis. This is done in the next
section by testing the effect of changing the mean and the
parameters of the requirement distribution on the estimate
of prevalence.

EFFECT OF REQUIREMENT DISTRIBUTION ON ESTIMATES OF THE
PREVALENCE OF INTAKE ADEQUACY

Influence of Mean and Standard Deviation of Requirement

NFCS data on vitamin C intake of adult men can be used
to illustrate how changes in the mean and the variability
of the requirement distribution can affect estimates of
the prevalence of inadequate intake. To account for changes
in the mean requirement, several hypothetical estimates of

the mean requirement of vitamin C are used, ranging from 10 mg/day to 60 mg/day. To explore the effect of changes in variability of requirement on the estimates, standard deviation estimates of 2, 4, 6, 8, and 10 mg/day were used, corresponding to coefficients of variation of 5%, 10%, 15%, 20%, and 25% where the mean requirement is 40 mg/day. Table 5-2 presents the results of probability analyses using each standard deviation estimate for each estimate of the mean requirement.

TABLE 5-2. Estimated Prevalence of Inadequate Vitamin C Intakes by Adult Males: An Illustration of the Sensitivity of the Probability Approach to the Mean and Variability of the Requirement Distribution[a]

Estimated Mean of the Requirement (mg/day)	Predicted Prevalence of Inadequate Intakes (%)[b] by SD of Requirement				
	SD[c] 2 mg/day	SD 4 mg/day	SD 6 mg/day	SD 8 mg/day	SD 10 mg/day
10	1.4	1.7	2.3	2.9	3.7
15	4.0	4.4	5.0	5.7	6.4
20	8.4	8.6	9.0	9.5	10.2
25	13.5	13.7	14.0	14.4	15.0
30	19.5	19.5	19.7	20.1	20.5
35	25.6	25.8	26.1	26.3	26.5
40	32.8	32.8	32.8	32.9	32.9
45	40.2	39.9	39.7	39.4	39.2
50	46.4	46.2	46.0	45.7	45.3
55	51.9	51.9	51.7	51.4	51.0
60	57.2	57.0	56.8	56.6	56.3

[a]Based on 1977-1978 NFCS data provided to the subcommittee.
[b]Inadequate is defined as an intake below requirement.
[c]Assumed standard deviation of the requirement distribution.

When mean requirement is held constant and the standard deviation is increased (across rows in Table 5-2), the predicted prevalence estimates do not change substantially. For example, for the estimated mean of 10 mg/day, the prevalence estimates range from 1.4% to 3.7%. For the highest mean of 60 mg/day, the prevalence estimate only changes from 57.2% to 56.3% at standard deviations of 2 and 10 mg/day, respectively. However, the prevalence estimates

are greatly affected by changes in the mean requirement,
as shown by comparing the estimates down the columns of
the table. For a standard deviation of 2 mg/day, the estimated prevalence of inadequate intake increases from 1.4%
for a requirement of 10 mg/day to 57.2% for a requirement
of 60 mg/day. This is generally true, regardless of the
estimated standard deviation. Thus, the prevalence of
inadequate intake is sensitive to the mean of the requirement distribution but is not greatly affected by the variance of the distribution.

Influence of the Shape of Requirement Distribution

Several nutrients were analyzed by the subcommittee to
determine how the shape of the distribution influences prevalence estimates. These analyses demonstrated that the
estimated prevalence is similar whether a normal assumption
is used or whether the probability of inadequacy is assumed
to increase in a linear manner. In this case, a probability of 0 was assigned to the mean requirement +2 SD, and a
probability of 1.0 was assigned to -2 SD.

The results of these analyses demonstrate empirically
that the model is not particularly sensitive to either the
variance of the requirement distribution or the shape of
the distribution, assuming that the requirement distribution is approximately symmetrical. For all nutrients
studied, the variability of the requirement appears to be
much smaller than the variability in the observed data on
nutrient intake. This is illustrated in Figure 5-3 in
which the probability curve is superimposed on the distribution of intakes. Generally, therefore, the errors of
overestimation and underestimation of the prevalence of
inadequate intake tend to cancel out, and except at the
ends of the intake distribution, the model is not sensitive to changes in the shape of the requirement distribution, i.e., its symmetry.

These empirical findings seem to apply to all the intake
distributions examined by the subcommittee (ascorbic acid,
protein, and vitamin A for adult males and females and
iron, thiamin, and thiamin/1,000 kcal for adult males),
assuming that requirements are distributed symmetrically
around the mean. When this condition is present, the
simplest empirical approach to estimating the prevalence
might be to determine the proportion of the study population with usual intakes below the mean requirement.

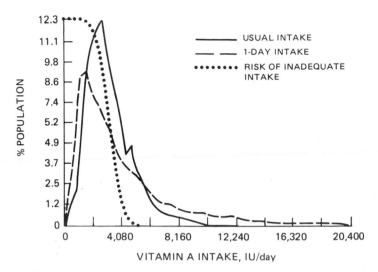

FIGURE 5-3.   One-day and adjusted distributions of vitamin A
             intake of adult females and superimposed proba-
             bility curve.   Note that the range in varia-
             tion of requirements is small in comparison to
             range of intakes.   It is assumed that require-
             ments are normally distributed with a 15% coef-
             ficient of variation.   Based on 1977-1978 NFCS
             data provided to the subcommittee.

Although this procedure will introduce some error into the
results, especially when the mean requirement is close to
the end of the intake distribution, the error is likely to
be within the confidence limits of the estimate.   For example, in the first row of Table 5-2, it would be difficult to
assert that 1.4% is different from 3.7%.   Conversely, one
might say with confidence that both are very low.   Thus, the
use of any reasonable standard deviation of requirement will
improve the estimate of prevalence.

The subcommittee also explored the use of the probability
approach when the requirement distribution is highly asymmetrical, e.g., for iron requirements of menstruating women.
(See Appendix B for the details of this analysis.)   The
relative shape of the curve is fixed by the known distribution of menstrual iron losses.   However, changing the
assumption about the upper limit of iron absorption will
also change the mean of the requirement distribution.   In
Table 5-3, prevalence has been estimated with the proba-

bility approach. It has also been estimated by using the logarithmic distribution of iron requirements and estimating the proportion of cases falling below the median require- ment. To change the position of the requirement distri- bution in this table, various iron absorption rates have been assumed. Iron absorption among women ingesting typical North-American mixed diets and maintaining iron stores has been estimated to be approximately 20% (FAO/WHO, 1970). Thus, the table compares two approaches to assessment across a family of requirement distributions.

When the requirement distribution is asymmetrical about the median, as it is for menstruating women, the propor- tion of persons falling below the median requirement is not a reliable estimate of the prevalence. (See last two col- umns of Table 5-3.) The full probability approach is manda- tory. The reason for this may be that unlike the vitamin A intake model in Figure 5-3, the range of the iron require- ment distribution encompasses a substantial part of the range of the dietary intake distribution. Because of the asymmetry of the requirement distribution, errors of under- and overestimation on the two sides of the median require-

TABLE 5-3. Comparison of Probability Estimates of the Prevalence of Inadequate Iron Intake and the Proportion of Intakes Falling Below the Mean Requirement[a]

Assumed Limit of Absorption (%)	Inferred Median Requirement (mg/day)[b]	Estimates Derived from Probability Approach	Estimates Derived Using Median Require- ment as Cutoff Point (%)
14	9.39	50.4	44.0
16	8.22	38.7	29.2
18	7.30	29.7	18.2
20	6.57	23.0	12.7
22	5.98	18.0	8.5
24	5.48	14.3	6.1
25	5.26	12.8	5.2

[a]Based on 1977-1978 NFCS data for menstruating women provided to the subcommittee.
[b]In the requirement distribution model used, the median physiological loss of iron is 1.32 mg/day.

ment would not be expected to cancel each other out. For iron, both the mean and the shape of the requirement distribution are important. For this reason, the simplified empirical approach in which the proportion below the median is used as an estimate of the prevalence of inadequacy cannot be applied to iron intake in menstruating women--or to any other nutrient where there is reason to believe that there is strong asymmetry in the distribution.

Impact of the Mode in Which Requirements Are Expressed

It is generally accepted that nutrient requirement estimates, and hence approaches to estimating the prevalence of inadequate intakes, must take into account the physiological variables of age, sex, pregnancy, and lactation. However, other variables that affect nutrient requirement should also be taken into account.

Current nutrient requirement reports (FAO/WHO/UNU, in press; Health and Welfare, Canada, 1983; NRC, 1980) recognize that body weight affects protein requirement. The primary requirement estimate is usually expressed as grams of protein per kilogram of body weight per day. Similarly, energy intake affects thiamin requirements, which are usually stated as mg/1,000 kcal/day. In addition, at least one report (Health and Welfare, Canada, 1983) recognizes the influence of protein intake on vitamin B_6 requirement, which is given as grams of protein intake per day.

In those reports, estimates are often applied to a representative subject to derive an estimate of recommended intake per day, without reference to the original variable that affected the requirement. This practice creates two potential problems. First, the variance of requirement per day may have been underestimated in this derivation. For example, if the variability of requirement for protein per kilogram of body weight has a CV of 15%, and this estimate must be extended to adult men, the variability of their body weights must be considered. The variability of protein requirement per day must be greater than that for protein requirement per kilogram of body weight per day (FAO/WHO/ UNU, in press). There are analogous situations for thiamin and vitamin B_6 requirements. To estimate prevalence, this adjustment of variance should be taken into account. However, since the final estimates of prevalence are not seriously affected by the magnitude of the variance of the requirement, this may not be a serious problem.

The second problem is much more important. If the variable of requirement (body weight, energy intake, or protein intake, in the examples cited above) is also associated with dietary intake of the nutrient, then there will be a spurious correlation between requirement per day and intake per day. A large man, for example, can be expected to have a higher protein requirement than a small man and is likely also to have a higher total food intake. In addition, protein intake is likely to be larger, resulting in a correlation between intake and requirement, unless body size is controlled. This contradicts a basic assumption underlying the probability approach, i.e., that there is a very low correlation between intake and requirement. The simplest way to avoid this is to express both requirement and intake in relation to common variables, e.g., per kilogram of body weight, per 1,000 kcal, or per gram of protein intake, as appropriate.

The impact of mode of expression on prevalence estimates for thiamin is shown numerically in Table 5-4. The two estimates of prevalence presented were both derived with the probability approach. One is based on an estimate of thiamin requirement per day. The other is based on an estimate of thiamin requirement per 1,000 kcal/day. Table 5-4 demonstrates that there is a substantial difference between the estimates derived in these two ways because in the second approach correlation between intake and requirement is avoided and there is recognition that a person with a low thiamin intake may also have a low energy intake and, hence, a low but adequate requirement for thiamin. In the 1980 Recommended Dietary Allowances, the proposed thiamin allowance was expressed as 0.5 mg/1,000 kcal/day (NRC, 1980). The average requirement was not explicitly stated, but the text implies that it is approximately 0.4 mg/1,000 kcal/day, with an implied CV of about 12.5%. In translating these into intakes per day, the Committee on Dietary Allowances assumed an average energy intake of about 3,000 kcal/day for the young adult male and derived an RDA of 1.5 mg/day. The imputed average requirement would be approximately 1.2 mg/day. Two different expressions of requirement distributions can be made: 0.4 ± 0.05 mg/1,000 kcal/day and 1.2 ± 0.15 mg/day. The effects of these two requirement estimates on the NFCS data are given in Table 5-4. The Committee on Dietary Allowances suggested that the relationship of thiamin requirement to energy intake may not be consistent at levels of energy intake, specifically less than 2,000 kcal/day. The modes of expression given in Table 5-4 do not take this RDA into account.

TABLE 5-4. Comparison of Two Approaches to the Assessment
of Thiamin Intake for Adult Males[a]

Mode of Expression of Intake and Requirement Data	Percentage of Population Predicted to Have Intakes Below Actual Requirements
mg/1,000 kcal/day	3.4
mg/day	36.9

[a]Based on data from 1977-1978 NFCS provided to the
subcommittee.

As illustrated by the analysis of thiamin, when a known
variable of requirement can be measured and applied in analysis, it is correct to express both intake and requirement
in relation to this variable before applying the probability approach to assessment, if fully valid prevalence estimates are to be obtained.

Impact of Criteria for Requirement Estimate

As discussed earlier, the criteria that serve as the
conceptual framework for the requirement estimate have a substantial effect on estimates of the prevalence of inadequate
intake. Two examples illustrate this principle. After examining the literature, an FAO/WHO committee (FAO/WHO, 1970)
concluded that an ascorbic acid intake of 10 mg/day was more
than minimally adequate to prevent or cure scurvy in adult
men. Since the range of requirements for this criterion of
adequacy appeared to be 6 to 10 mg/day, one might assume a
mean requirement of 8 mg/day and a CV of 15%. The Committee
on Dietary Allowances agreed with this estimate of the
requirement to prevent scurvy; however, it accepted metabolic pool size as the basis for deriving the recommended
allowance and suggested that the upper tail of the requirement range, the recommended intake, was approximately 60
mg/day (NRC, 1980). That committee's report suggests that
the CV of this requirement might be 15% to 20%. Estimates
of the requirement distribution for the maintenance of an
adequate body pool can be derived as a mean requirement of
45 mg/day with a CV of 15%. Using this logic, one can define
two different criteria for vitamin C requirement distributions, and the results obtained with these two different criteria can be compared. To explore their impact on the preva-

lence of inadequate intake, these two requirement distributions were applied to NFCS data. The resulting estimates of
inadequate intake for vitamin C are shown in Table 5-5.

In 1963, a committee (Health and Welfare, Canada, 1964)
reviewed the evidence and concluded that a thiamin intake of
0.2 mg/1,000 kcal/day was adequate to prevent clinical signs
of beriberi in adults. An FAO/WHO (1967) committee cited
evidence suggesting that 0.23 mg/1,000 kcal was higher than
the requirement that would prevent any functional aberration
for at least 12 weeks. In the United States, the Committee
on Dietary Allowances (NRC, 1980) suggested that even lower
levels might be adequate to prevent beriberi. Making a
judgment based on these three estimates, the present subcommittee estimated that the average thiamin requirement for
the prevention of clinically detectable malfunction is
approximately 0.2 mg/1,000 kcal per day, with a CV of about
15%. However, none of the committees believed that this
requirement was desirable for maintenance of a suitable
state of health, and all of them estimated requirements on
the basis of metabolic function or implied tissue levels.
For example, the Committee on Dietary Allowances (NRC, 1980)
recommended an intake of 0.5 mg/1,000 kcal/day but did not
specify the underlying requirement distribution. To illustrate the importance of changes in nutrient requirement, an

TABLE 5-5.   Prevalence of Inadequate Intake Estimated
               with Two Different Assumptions About
               Requirement Distributions of Adult Men[a]

Criterion of Adequacy for Requirement	Estimated Prevalence of Inadequate Intakes (%)	
	Ascorbic Acid	Thiamin[b]
Avoidance of clinically detectable malfunction	0.7	0
Maintenance of tissue levels or metabolic pools	39.6	3.4

[a]Based on 1977-1978 NFCS data provided to the
subcommittee.
[b]Thiamin intakes per 1,000 kcal examined. No lower
limit was placed on absolute level of thiamin intake.

average requirement of 0.4 mg/day with a CV of approximately 12.5% can be used. The prevalence of inadequate thiamin intake was determined for each of these two criteria as given in Table 5-5.

As shown in Table 5-5, estimates of the prevalence of inadequate intake depend on the criterion of nutritional adequacy underlying the requirement estimate. Agreement between the dietary assessment and a biochemical or clinical assessment of the same population depends to a large extent on both the concordance between the underlying concepts of adequacy that have been used to set the dietary requirement and the biochemical or clinical criterion. Not surprisingly, current approaches often result in different estimates of the prevalence of inadequate nutrition when the same criterion of adequacy has not been used to establish requirements for dietary intake and criteria for biochemical measurements.

Comparison with Fixed Cutoff Approach

In Table 5-6, prevalence estimates derived with the probability approach are compared with those based on the fixed cutoff approach. The bases of the probability estimates were presented earlier in this chapter. Four arbitrary cutoff points, expressed as percentages of the RDA (NRC, 1980), have been used.

TABLE 5-6. Comparison of Estimates of the Prevalence of Inadequate Intakes for Adults Using Probability and Fixed Cutoff Approaches[a]

Nutrient and Sex Group	Prevalence Estimates(%), by Approach Used				
	Probability Approach	Fixed Cutoff Approach			
		100% RDA	80% RDA	70% RDA	60% RDA
Protein (males)	2.3	6.5	2.4	1.3	0.8
Vitamin C (males)	39.6	57.5	44.5	36.3	27.1
Iron (females)	23.0	98.2	91.2	81.6	62.5

[a]Applied to adjusted data from 1977-1978 NFCS provided to the subcommittee.

It becomes immediately apparent from the table that a fixed cutoff approach may or may not give estimates of the prevalence of inadequate intakes similar to those generated with the probability approach. However, the cutoff point that produces the similarity is specific to the characteristics of both the requirement distribution and intake distribution. Thus it may or may not be correct. For this reason, analysis of prevalence with cutoff points is not recommended.

The possibility of using the mean nutrient requirement as a cutoff point was also considered by the subcommittee. This would be a possible alternative if the following conditions apply: the requirement distribution is reasonably symmetrical, the mean requirement does not fall in the tail of the intake distribution, and the variance of dietary intake is greater than the variance of the requirement for that nutrient.

SUMMARY

When the shape of the distribution of nutrient requirement is known or can be inferred, a probability approach to the assessment of observed nutrient intakes is the most efficient and logical analytical approach. If, as is a reasonable assumption for most nutrients, the requirements are distributed relatively symmetrically about the mean or median, the probability approach is sensitive to the estimate of the average requirement. It is, however, relatively insensitive to the shape and variance of the requirement distribution in the assessment of population data.

6

Assessing Excessive Intake and Nutrient Energy Ratios

Excessive intake can present serious health problems. The subcommittee therefore discussed factors of major concern with regard to overconsumption and explored the use of the probability approach to assess excessive intakes.

FAT INTAKE

Approaches to adjusting the distribution of observed intakes to estimate the distribution of usual intakes can be applied to fats, which are of concern because of a possible effect of high intakes on serum lipids and coronary heart disease. Through the use of such approaches, subgroups can be compared or trends examined over time. Moreover, the distribution of intakes can be compared with recommended intakes promulgated by various groups. This technique may also be adequate for establishing whether overall population intakes should be increased or decreased. It would be desirable to assess prevalence of excess fat intake in such a manner in light of current concerns.

Present knowledge is inadequate for the subcommittee to offer specific guidance on assessing the intake of fat. However, it has considered a construct for assessing excessive intake of fat, carbohydrate, or indeed any nutrient. This construct, which is presented later in this chapter, can be used when data portraying the probability of excessive intake have been assembled in a manner similar to that used to assess probability of inadequate intake.

41

NONNUTRIENTS

The U.S. public's interest in nutrition appears to have shifted in recent years from concern only about deficiency diseases to concern about both inadequate consumption and overconsumption. The number of dietary components of interest has also grown from only those whose intake is required for good health to those whose intake is somehow related to maintenance of optimal health. Included in the latter are nonnutritive compounds that are related to the onset and development of such diseases as cancer and cardiovascular disease. Many of these compounds have not traditionally been listed in food composition tables. The subcommittee suggests that future tables include listings of the concentrations of those compounds known to enhance or retard the development of chronic diseases. It believes that such additions to the food composition tables will significantly enhance the ability of the USDA to respond to anticipated questions from the U.S. public about the intake of food components and will provide the U.S. population with much better information on the adequacy and safety of its diet.

Assessment of the Prevalence of Excessive Intake

In Chapter 5, the probability approach was discussed in relation to estimating the prevalence of inadequate nutrient intake. The main feature of this approach is its recognition of requirement variations among similar individuals that are taken into account in estimating the probability of adequacy of a particular intake level and generalizing to the population or subpopulation by summing the estimates of prevalence for each intake level.

The same principles and approach can be used to analyze detrimentally high usual intakes of nutrients or food components. The risk of acute toxicity cannot be estimated in this fashion from survey dietary intake data. Individual variation in response to a detrimental factor is analogous to the variability of nutrient requirement, which has already been discussed. If a mean level of excess intake can be derived, it can be analyzed with a probability approach similar to the analysis of mean requirement. Thus, a distribution of intakes that would be deemed excessive can be conceptualized. If this distribution can be described or estimated, the probability approach can be applied in the same manner as described for inadequate intake, except that attention will be focused on the upper end of the adjusted intake distribution and the lower end of the requirement distributions.

The concepts embodied in this approach have been presented by two recent committees dealing with nutrient requirements (FAO/WHO/UNU, in press; Health and Welfare, Canada, 1983) and are illustrated in Figure 6-1. The left-hand curve of this figure is identical in concept and derivation to the curve presented in Figure 5-1 to portray the probability of inadequacy of protein intake. In Figure 6-1, the recommended intake is marked on the curve indicating the level of intake associated with a very low probability of inadequacy for a randomly selected member of the population. The curve on the right is meant to portray the analogous probability that a particular level of intake will be detrimental to the randomly selected individual. A point marking low risk is shown. Both this point and the recommended intake might be considered safe, i.e., intakes representing an acceptably

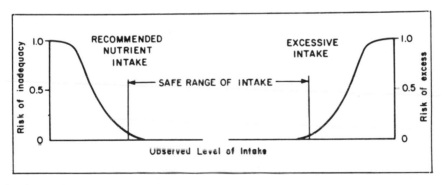

FIGURE 6-1.   The concept of a safe intake range. Since there is individual variability in both requirement for a nutrient and tolerance for high usual intake, the risk or probability curves for inadequacy and for excess may be described as in Figure 5-1. The safe intake range is associated with a very low probability of either inadequacy or excess for an individual selected at random from the population. From Health and Welfare, Canada, 1983.

low risk or probability of either inadequacy or detrimental
excess. The range of intakes falling between these two
points can be regarded as a safe range of intakes for individuals. By altering the definition of acceptable risk or
probability, the range will be extended or contracted.

Two implications and applications of these concepts are
relevant to the present report. Consider first the presence of detrimental factors in foods. By using the right-
hand curve, it is theoretically possible to estimate the
prevalence of excess intakes in a manner directly parallel
to that described for estimating the prevalence of inadequate intakes. Adjustment of intake distributions to elim-
inate the effects of day-to-day variation would be carried
out in the same manner as described above. The prerequi-
site for applying the probability approach would be a
description of, or judgment about, the frequency distribution of intakes that are detrimental for individuals in the
population. The application of the probability approach in
this area of research is at present constrained by the
lack of attention to the examination of this distribution.
Bearing in mind this constraint, the subcommittee recognizes
that the probability approach can be used for excessive
intakes as well as inadequate intakes whenever there is sufficient information on the distribution of excess intakes.

The approach can also be used to assess the appropri-
ateness of nutrient intake when there is reason for concern about both inadequate and excessive intake. A specific and important example would be the assessment of fat
intake in the NFCS survey. On one hand, inadequate intake
of fat or fatty acids can result in specific fatty acid
deficiencies and too low an energy density in the diet.
On the other hand, excess fat intake can produce detrimental effects on serum lipids and has been implicated
in the development of atherosclerosis. To determine the
optimal level of fat intake for a population, one should
take into account both risk curves portrayed in Figure 6-1.
The application of this type of analysis in nutrition
programming would logically be directed toward the encour-
agement of dietary intake within the safe intake range.
This assessment is limited, however, by the absence of
descriptions of the distributions of intake levels that
would be inadequate or excessive--the two requirement distributions. Before there can be any scientific approach
to the assessment of biologically appropriate or safe
intake levels, these curves must be defined.

ENERGY FROM PROTEIN, FAT, AND CARBOHYDRATE

A technical approach to defining criteria for protein-to-energy ratios has been presented by the Committee on Energy and Protein Requirements of FAO/WHO/UNU (in press). This approach requires knowledge of the distribution of protein requirements, of energy requirements, and of the correlation between the two. The same technical approach could be applied to fat and carbohydrate, if requirement distributions become known (FAO/WHO/UNU, in press).

The major problem in applying nutrient energy ratios is that the distribution of energy requirements changes with the distribution of physical activity characteristic of the population or population subgroup (FAO/WHO/UNU, in press). In theory, this might mean that a distribution of the ratio of nutrient to energy requirements (nutrient density) should be determined for each population subgroup based on a distribution of energy requirements for that subpopulation. For this reason, the subcommittee sees no advantage in assessing the biological suitability of observed nutrient density in population studies of dietary intake and offers no guidelines for this type of evaluation, because more information about requirements is required to apply this approach than for the probability approach.

The concept of nutrient density, which relates nutrients to energy or volume of food, may be useful for other purposes, such as in considering the nutritional quality of individual foods or in providing prescriptive recommendations for diet modifications. For community diagnoses or needs assessment, however, there is no apparent advantage to examining nutrient-to-energy ratios rather than nutrient intake, except when energy is a determinant of requirement for a nutrient as for thiamin. These other applications of nutrient density ratios do not fall within the scope of the mandate assigned to the subcommittee.

If it can be assumed that activity levels and anthropometric status are to remain constant, the distribution of usual energy intake is taken to describe approximately the distribution of energy requirements. If, however, observed energy intake describes the distribution of energy requirement, there will be no purpose to the use of this information for population assessment since this same distribution serves as the intake distribution. The final assessment would be identical with that obtained by assessing observed protein intake per kilogram of body weight. Although the same principles would hold for assessment of energy derived from fats or carbohydrates, the situation is more difficult because no descriptors of the requirement distribution are available.

In view of the other uses of nutrient density information and the increasing popularity of this method of describing the diet of a population, the subcommittee recognizes that the USDA may wish to publish descriptive information about the energy derived from fat, carbohydrate, and protein. For this purpose it suggests that centile distribution may be appropriate. Such centile distributions should only be generated after the intake distributions have been adjusted to remove the effects of day-to-day variations.

The interpretation of such information in relation to epidemiological studies or similar studies requires caution, because fats, protein and carbohydrates together with alcohol make up the total energy intake, and if the intake of one decreases there must be compensatory increases in the intake of one or more of the others. To interpret such information, one should take into account the covariances among these macronutrients, which will not be apparent from simple centile distributions of the individual macronutrient-to-energy ratios.

USE OF THE PROBABILITY APPROACH TO ASSESS ENERGY INTAKE

As was discussed in Chapter 3, the probability approach to analyzing dietary adequacy requires either a knowledge of the joint distribution of dietary intake and requirement or an assumption of independence. For the nutrients, it is reasonable to assume that intake is determined to a very large extent by psychosocial factors affecting the selection of particular foods rather than by physiological factors. Studies in animal models indicate, however, that there are specific regulatory mechanisms for nutrient intake and provide limited evidence that these mechanisms continue to operate as an important factor in determining nutrient intake by free-living subjects. Therefore, it is reasonable to assume independence of intake and requirement for nutrients, provided the obvious factors affecting both intake and requirement (e.g., age, sex, and major differences in body size) have been taken into account.

Energy intake and expenditure are highly correlated among individuals, and regulatory mechanisms adjust intake to expenditure or adjust expenditure to intake (FAO/WHO/UNU, in press). The probability approach cannot be used to assess dietary energy intake and to interpret NFCS data on energy intake until specific knowledge has accrued on the magnitude of this correlation. In the assessment of dietary adequacy, therefore, energy intake must be interpreted in a manner completely different from that used for nutrient intake data.

For example, since activity is a major variable of energy expenditure, observed energy intake may be used as a descriptor of the usual expenditure levels and of status quo activity levels (Beaton, 1983). Examination of the energy status of a population requires measures of energy stores, such as anthropometric measurements, which are collected in the United States by the National Health and Nutrition Examination Survey.

7

Errors in Nutrient Intake Measurement

All measurements have components of random errors and systematic bias. Dietary intake measurements are no exception. In developing an approach to the analysis of dietary data, it is essential to consider the effect of both types of error. The estimates of nutrient intake are based on data from dietary surveys, data in food composition tables, and the computation of the nutrient intake from these two data sets. Each data set has sources of random error and bias; there is also potential for bias in the computation process. Thus, the subcommittee discussed sources of bias and variability in the data on dietary intake, food composition, and computation of nutrient intake. This chapter presents the results of its analysis of the impact of random error and systematic bias on the estimates of the prevalence of inadequate intake.

SAMPLING VARIATION

Random Error

By chance, the persons randomly selected in dietary surveys may not be representative of the reference population. Using statistical theory, one can derive minimum estimates of this sampling error, which would be increased by other sources of variability such as those discussed in this chapter.

Systematic Bias

Systematic bias in sampling can also occur. For example, in such surveys as the Nationwide Food Consumption Survey (NFCS), the sample design is based on households. Therefore, the homeless are systematically underrepresented. Self-selection (i.e., survey participation by consent) can also produce an unrepresentative sample of the U.S. population and result in systematic bias. When there are several components to the collection of data, fewer persons may respond in one component than in another. For example, fewer persons may complete dietary diaries than respond to a household interview. This bias would be especially problematic if those who completed diaries were better organized and better educated than those who were only interviewed. The magnitude of bias from sample design and from nonresponse requires special research not usually included in surveys of this kind. At a minimum, it is important to determine the probable direction of any such bias and, where possible, it is preferable to estimate the magnitude as well.

ERRORS IN ESTIMATING USUAL NUTRIENT INTAKE

Errors in Reporting Usual Food Intake

Day-to-Day Variation in Intake. The intake of concern is the average intake of individuals across time. This usual intake is believed to affect tissue levels of the nutrients and body functions. Intake on a particular day does not reliably portray the usual intake.

The impact of day-to-day variation in intake is discussed in some detail in Chapter 4, where the subcommittee discusses a method to adjust dietary intake to control for day-to-day variation. Although several statistical techniques might be used for this purpose, the subcommittee chose to use an analysis of variance procedure for the analyses presented in this report.

Variability in Reporting and Recording Food Intake. A close examination of errors in reporting, recording, and coding data from food intake surveys is helpful in identifying errors that are random within a person and those that are systematic.

● Random error. A respondent may sometimes overreport and sometimes underreport in a random fashion. Variation also occurs between persons when one person underreports and another person overreports. Even if these errors are random, they present a problem in the analysis of population data. However, systematic bias involving entire subgroups of the population may have more serious implications for the analysis of such data. For example, if all or most members of the lower socioeconomic groups overestimate intake of such status foods as meat, biased estimates of iron intake may result.

• Systematic bias. In the NFCS, the importance of systematic underreporting in the total population has been recognized. As a result, the U.S. Department of Agriculture (USDA) has undertaken or funded numerous studies that address these problems. The literature relating to these questions is reviewed briefly in the following paragraphs.

The goal of any dietary survey is to measure what people eat--more precisely, to measure what foods and supplements people habitually eat or usually ingest. Dietary survey methods can be classified into two general categories: methods based on memory (recall) and methods based on records. In memory-based procedures, subjects are asked to recall all food and drink consumed over a specified time, usually 24 hours. Record-keeping methods take several forms: a common procedure is to ask subjects to keep a diary recording all foods and beverages consumed during a specified number of days, most commonly for periods of up to 7 days. In some cases, respondents are provided with plastic or paper food models and measuring devices to aid in estimating portion sizes. In other cases, they receive only specific written or oral instructions or both. As mentioned earlier, the recall and record methods were combined in the collection of 3-day dietary intake data for individuals in the 1977-1978 NFCS.

In recent years there have been several reviews of dietary methods (Beal and Laus, 1982; Becker et al., 1960; Burk and Pao, 1976; Marr, 1971) as well as many papers concerned with the quality of specific methods. The aspect of quality of greatest concern is validity, especially with regard to systematic bias in data on dietary intake.

A valid method is one that measures what it intends to measure--the true intake of subjects. Dietary methods can be validated only by knowledge of true intake or by some sensitive laboratory measurement of intake. Block (1982) notes that it is difficult to ascertain true

intake over long periods. Consequently, validation frequently consists of comparing one dietary survey method
with another. Such validation is limited by the lack of
agreement on a "true" or reference method. Similarities
in the two methods may fail to detect common errors when
the two methods are compared. Failure to record accurately all foods eaten during a survey may influence subsequent recall. It may also sensitize the respondent's
power of observation, so that a subsequent recall is more
complete than the initial daily record, as in a survey or
nutritional assessment.

Unobtrusive observations of actual intake have been
made of people in various institutional settings, such as
children in grade schools (Comstock et al., 1981; Graves
and Shannon, 1983; Lachance, 1976; Meredith et al., 1951),
students in college cafeterias (Krantzler et al., 1982;
Mullen et al., 1984; Raker, 1979), elderly people at con-
gregate meal settings (Gersovitz et al., 1978; Madden et
al., 1976), patients in nursing homes (Caliendo, 1981),
adolescents in a metabolic research unit (Greger and
Etnyre, 1978), young boys consuming food at home for a
1-day period (Stunkard and Waxman, 1981), lactating women
confined to a hospital (Linusson et al., 1975), and
massively obese patients in a clinical research center
(Bray et al., 1978). Settings such as these are optimal
for these studies because portions served are standard-
ized or predetermined. These observations have usually
been made for short periods or even for single meals,
although observations as long as 28 consecutive days were
reported by Mullen et al. (1984) and Krantzler et al.
(1982) in their study of students in a dormitory dining
hall. Institutional routines may, however, alter the
eating patterns and recall as compared to the general
population.

Caveats about validation must be taken into account
before the accuracy and systematic bias in food intake
data are addressed. For example, are there systematic
errors in the dietary intakes reported by some subgroups
of the population, such as young and old subjects, or in
the reporting of particular foods or food groups--biases
that would influence the reported nutrient intakes?

The results of several validation studies indicate that
low intakes may be overreported and high intakes underreported, with a resultant flat-slope syndrome (Gersovitz

et al., 1978; Madden et al., 1976; Stunkard and Waxman, 1981), although mean intakes for groups may be accurately recalled. However, the flat slope syndrome may be nothing more than the attenuation of the slope that arises from random error in the independent variable, as has been described by many authors.

Systematic biases may exist in dietary reporting by selected population subgroups but have not been sufficiently addressed to warrant conclusions. For example, Campbell and Dodds (1967) used a 24-hour recall to collect dietary information from elderly and young patients hospitalized for various lung disorders. Their purpose was to test the extent of error when a 24-hour recall was used to collect information from elderly subjects whose failing memory may affect recall. The 24-hour recall data were checked by prompting subjects based on a known menu. In this study, the elderly subjects underreported calories more often than did younger subjects, and men underreported more calories than did women. Dietary intakes obtained without probing were approximately 25% lower than those obtained with probing.

Marr (1971) concluded that it is difficult to obtain valid dietary data from young children. For example, it is necessary to rely on a surrogate, such as a parent, to provide information about the intake of young children. In addition, caretakers other than parents frequently provide food for the child, making it difficult to secure the necessary data. In the United States, food is increasingly eaten away from home by young children as more and more preschoolers attend childcare facilities.

A preliminary study of 29 children of preschool age was designed to examine the relative usefulness of the 1-day food record and the 24-hour recall (H. Smiciklas-Wright and P. Holmberg, Pennsylvania State University, personal communication, 1985). The investigators observed actual intake at a lunch consumed by children attending a day-care center and then asked 14 mothers to provide data on dietary intake by a 24-hour recall. Seven of the 14 mothers provided no data for the meals consumed while their children were at the center. The remaining mothers failed to identify menu items correctly, overestimated portion sizes, or both. The 15 parents who provided information by a 1-day record did provide more complete data, although these parents also tended to misidentify foods or overestimate portion sizes. For data interpretation it is important to know whether a surrogate reporter was present at all meals.

Retrospective diet histories have been compared with direct measurements of food intake by obese patients hospitalized in a metabolic unit (Bray et al., 1978). Three retrospective assessments of diet history were obtained at 1-month intervals. In the first history, energy intake was underestimated. By the third one, estimates of energy intake had risen—particularly because of improved reporting of alcohol intake. Thus, the third history probably provided the best correlation between true and reported energy intake.

Lansky and Brownell (1982) also examined the accuracy of food records of applicants in a behavioral weight-reduction program. Thirty women estimated the quantity of 10 foods that were displayed in small and large containers. Container size did not influence quantity estimates, but the quantities of all 10 foods were over-estimated. The amount of overestimation varied from a small overestimation for cola and orange juice to a large overestimation for potato chips, ham, and turkey. Neither Bray et al. (1978) nor Lansky and Brownell (1982) reported comparable data on subjects of normal weight to determine whether the errors in reporting intake and recording serving sizes were restricted to obese persons. A. Blake (Pennsylvania State University, personal communication, 1985) found that serving sizes were underestimated by both obese subjects and persons within normal weight ranges. This investigator provided preweighed portions of foods at a lunch attended by subjects who were contacted the next day for a 24-hour recall. The majority of subjects, both obese and normal, underestimated the servings they had eaten.

Sopko et al. (1984) found that obese males reported from 78% to 93% of their actual intake in a controlled feeding experiment. Although the study was not a true validation, Hallfrisch et al. (1982) observed that on a 7-day diet record, men reported 80% and women reported 65% of the consumed calories in subsequent 6-week experimental periods.

These results call into question the validity of recall or recording of food intake. Reports of food and energy intakes only slightly higher than basal energy requirements of adult women are difficult to reconcile with population data showing a 40% prevalence of overweight and a 25.7% prevalence of obesity, as indicated by body mass index (Van Itallie and Woteki, 1985).

Selective underreporting is also suggested by comparisons of beer, wine, and distilled spirit consumption, as reported for adult males and females in the NFCS and National Health and Nutrition Examination Survey (NHANES), to estimates of alcohol disappearance, as reported by the Bureau of Alcohol, Firearms, and Tobacco Control (Pao et al., 1982). Similarly, Schnakenberg et al. (1981), studying the reported food intake of 62 men in a military dining hall for a 7-day period in comparison to observed and weighed intakes, found that 13% underestimated their caloric intake by more than 30% and 34% underestimated their caloric intake by 10% to 20%. Only 5% overestimated by more than 30%.

In contrast, de St. Jeor (1980), who monitored weight status to validate the accuracy of energy intake reported by paid, educated subjects over a 12-week period, concluded that recorded intakes were an acceptable measure of actual intake. As reported earlier, A. Blake (Pennsylvania State University, personal communication, 1985), comparing the recalled intake of meals to observed and weighed intakes by obese and nonobese subjects, found no difference between the two groups, but did confirm a tendency to overreport small intakes and underreport higher intakes. She found estimated portion sizes to vary from actual sizes by less than 10% for most food items.

One reason for the discrepancy between actual and reported intake may be the difficulty that respondents have in estimating portion sizes. Guthrie (1984) found that for 13 food items, from 6% to 75% of adult male and female subjects reported portion sizes that varied by more than 50% from the weighed portion sizes. However, only 26% of the respondents consistently under- or overreported all items in the meal. H. Smiciklas-Wright and H. Guthrie (Pennsylvania State University, personal communication, 1984) showed that the ability of college-age students to estimate within 1 oz the volume of fluid contained in drinking glasses varied from 30% to 70%, depending on the size and shape of the container.

Young et al. (1952) found that for a variety of foods the direction of error was generally in overestimating por-

tions. Compensations were made for this bias by using zero
for all omissions of data when calculating means. They concluded that for the group, errors in the estimation of portion sizes for most food types are probably within 20% of
actual portions, except for children's recall, which has a
greater error.

Krantzler et al. (1982) reported on 24-hour recall and 3-
day or 7-day records of students who were observed periodically over a 28-day period during which they took their
meals in a dormitory dining hall. They reported that foods
eaten regularly, i.e., those contributing the major part of
a meal, were better reported than such foods as condiments,
nuts, and seeds. Estimates of dairy products, meat, and
fish were the most accurate. Guthrie (1984) reported that
few subjects in her study forgot main meal items, but one
in six respondents forgot to mention salad dressing.
Because two-thirds of the respondents used more than 20 g
(about 130 kcal) of salad dressing, that omission alone
could represent a sizable error in daily intake.

The foregoing discussion suggests that errors in
reporting dietary intake undoubtedly exist. The studies
suggest also that the direction of errors varies from study
to study and perhaps from population group to popu- lation
group. In a separate exercise, the committee com- pared
the distributions of intakes reported in several recent
large surveys. There were differences, suggesting bias in
either estimation of food intake or food composition data, but these were not consistent across nutrients.
The evidence is not sufficiently consistent to suggest how
these systematic biases affect estimates of individual
nutrients. It is clear, however, that they can do so
markedly. Because the 1977-1978 NFCS did not include data
on nutrient supplements, it certainly underestimated the
intake.

Variability Due to Coding and Analysis of the Nutrient Content of Foods

Sources of Technical Errors in Food Composition. The
technical errors in food composition data that influence
the interpretation of food consumption surveys fall into
three broad categories: true random variability of the
composition of individual food items, biased food composition data, and the differences in bioavailability of
individual dietary nutrients.

● <u>True random variability</u>. Variations in the composition of a food item from the population mean as given
in their classification codes reflects the true variation
in nutrient content of foods due to differences in produc-
tion practices and to the effects on raw materials exerted
by such variables as soil, fertilizer application, weather,
pest control, and genetic variation. Postharvest physiological changes, storage, and processing also contribute
to the true variability of the nutrient content of individual foods.

Estimates of this normal variation were included in the
current USDA food composition data tables, which were used
for the sensitivity analysis of dietary intake information
included later in this chapter. This analysis indicates
that normal food composition variation contributes a
significant portion of the total variation in the
estimated intake of given nutrients. However, the subcommittee suspects that an all-out effort to decrease the
standard error of the mean of the data in the food
composition data base is not needed in most cases. Even
though food composition contributes to variation, coefficients of variation due to errors in the computation of
intakes for most nutrients are generally small and the
overall error is modest. The subcommittee suggests that
sensitivity analysis be applied to the specific nutrients
to determine the effect of reducing the error of the mean.
The results of the sensitivity analysis should then be
used to develop priorities designating which nutrients
require further refinements either by assaying more samples or developing more precise analytical methodology.

● <u>Biased food composition data</u>. Errors in food
composition data result when the data are consistently
incorrect due to the methods of data collection or analysis. Often neither the direction nor extent of bias is
known for individual foods. Common causes of biased data
are incorrect identification of the food item, the use of
inappropriate analytical methodology, and the use of imputed
values. Incorrect identification of the food being analyzed, despite the precision of the analytical technique
used in the assay, leads to biased data. Thus, the subcommittee encourages the USDA to continue with its ongoing
efforts to improve the food nomenclature system.

The nutrient values in the current food composition data
bases for food categories are weighted averages of the con-

tents of the individual foods that fall within the category of the listing. Such data are acceptable for calculating nutrient intake if the nutrient content of each food is randomly distributed about the mean for the food category. In such cases the estimated nutrient intakes can be reasonably calculated from the mean content of the food category. However, the use of such mean values to estimate nutrient intake can lead to significant bias when the nutrient content of the food item is not randomly distributed about the mean of the food group.

For some categories of processed and manufactured foods, means are not representative of values for certain brands because their nutrient contents are controlled by recipes or processes with unique formulations significantly different from the category mean. Formulations vary to this extent for only some foods and even then for only some nutrients in those foods. For example, wide variations in nutrient content could be found in vitamin-fortified fruit juices and breakfast cereals, the sugar content of breakfast cereals, the fat content of bakery products, and the sodium content of many different prepared foods and meals. When brand loyalty is considerable, that is, when consumers consistently use the same brand rather than randomly selecting similar products, and when the mean nutrient content of the brand item differs from that of the category mean, biases will occur in the calculated estimations of nutrient intake. Such problems can be corrected by using brand-specific composition data. Since the addition of brand name identifiers may increase the complexity, and therefore the cost, of the food composition data and food consumption surveys, the subcommittee suggests that sensitivity analysis be used to determine which brands need to be identified by brand name to improve estimates of the intake of particular nutrients.

The analytical methods constitute a recognized source of bias in food composition data. In some cases, the methods do not measure all chemical forms of the nutrient, thus leading to underreporting for foods that contain the unmeasured chemical forms. Other nutrient assays are inhibited by some food components, and when such components are present, the nutrient content will be underreported. Certain assays respond to components other than the nutrient of interest, and when such substances are present, the nutrient content will be overreported.

Where there are no direct data on the nutrient composition of a particular food, nutrient values can be calculated by summing the contributions of each component of the formulation, if the food item is formulated from several other food components with known values. Although the resulting figures usually give acceptable estimates of the nutrient content of the foods, in some cases a value is imputed for the nutrient by using the nutrient content of a similar food and bias may be introduced. For example, lacking analytical values for corn syrup, known composition values for molasses might be imputed under the assumption that corn syrup had the same composition. This results in an overestimation of iron intake, because molasses contains a good deal of iron and commercial syrup has none. Imputed and calculated values in the current USDA food composition tables can be identified because the entry for the number of samples is left blank. However, there is no way for the users of the tables to determine directly if the other nutrient values are imputed or calculated.

The subcommittee recommends that the practice of imputing food composition values be avoided. When sensitivity analysis shows that imputing the content of certain foods may result in significant errors in estimating the prevalence of inadequate intake, the components of those foods must be analyzed. However, no person's dietary information should be omitted because there are no analyzed data for converting foods to nutrients. Thus, values for many foods must be imputed. It is important therefore that these imputations be reasonable estimates. For instance, assigning zero as an imputed value simply because the data are not available is not a reasonable estimate. If imputed values are used, they should be flagged so that their impact on the data analysis can be considered.

● Biases due to food composition data--incorrect assessment of differences in bioavailability of nutrients. The selection of criteria for assessing nutritional intake is complicated by the variation in absorption of nutrients. For example, evidence indicates that the bioavailability of iron varies with its chemical form in the diet (e.g., heme versus nonheme; reduced iron versus iron phosphates); the presence or absence of absorption enhancers in the meal (e.g., ascorbic acid or the "meat factor"); the presence or absence of compounds in the meal, such as phytates and tannic acid, which reduce the absorption of iron; and the physiological status of the small intestine as it relates to the state of the iron stores of the individual (Morris, 1983). The assessment of the iron intake of individuals has several components: the iron requirement of different age and sex groups, the food composition data, and often an assessment of the bioavailability of iron in the meals. To take into account the bioavailability of iron in the diet in the 1980 RDAs, a factor of 10 was applied to the actual requirement to account for absorption losses. In contrast, data based on food composition do not usually contain any direct information on the bioavailability of iron in individual foods. However, this is not always the case. For vitamin E, most food composition data bases do have a built-in estimate of bioavailability for each food. The subcommittee believes that inclusion of the bioavailability of iron in calculation of requirements introduces a potential source of bias in the assessment of nutrient intake. Some forms of iron are available at much less than the 10% level and some at higher levels. Although the use of a fixed level of absorption does not take into account the influence of the iron sources on its bioavailability, a 20% level has been suggested as the upper limit by an FAO/WHO (1970) committee and some of the calculations in this report are based on this limit (see Appendix B).

It is possible to improve the data on bioavailability by beginning with the actual requirement for absorbed iron for each age and sex category. This can be done by removing the correction factor for the lack of iron availability from the stated iron requirement). The concentrations of each chemical form of the iron in each food in the food composition data base can then be listed together with the concentrations of each iron absorption enhancer and inhibitor for each food in the data base. In this way it is possible to develop algorithms to calculate the biologically available iron for each meal based on the chemical form(s) of the enhancers and the inhibitors in the meal. Although this approach will provide a better estimate of the iron intake of individuals and thus populations, it requires the development of new computer algorithms. It thus requires more research, which must be guided by sensitivity analysis to avoid research and analysis of marginal utility.

Nutrient Data with Probable Bias

In a recent report of the National Research Council, the current status of the methodology for nutrient analysis in foods was discussed (NRC, 1984). Methods for assaying several of the nutrients of concern to this subcommittee were found to be less than adequate. In particular, the authors found that the methods for vitamin A, carotenoids, vitamin B_{12}, vitamin C, and folacin were such that there was only a fair probability that these methods would produce correct values. Following are detailed discussions of the status of these nutrients.

Vitamin A. Data on the composition of foods containing preformed vitamin A (whether naturally present or added during processing) appear to be reasonable, since the methods used to obtain them appear to be reasonable assay systems. Thus, the subcommittee believes that estimates of the dietary intake of vitamin A from these data are reasonable.

Carotenoids. Approximately 50 carotenoids possess vitamin A activity, each apparently with its own biological potency. Currently the vitamin A contributions of all these compounds are lumped together in food composition data bases as retinol equivalents. The chemical assay of the carotenoids is very complex (particularly in fruits and vegetables), and the current techniques used for food assay are not adequate for the determination of all the carotenoids in foods. Furthermore, there is no agreement on the assignment of biological potency as vitamin A for each carotenoid isomer. The subcommittee suggests that studies be undertaken to determine the concentration of each carotenoid isomer in fruits and vegetables. If such studies are undertaken, consideration should also be given to the concept of measuring all carotenoid isomers because of the interest in the apparent protective effects these may have as anticancer agents. There is no apparent reason to believe that only the carotenoids with vitamin A activity may have anticancer activity.

Vitamin B_{12}. The current acceptable assay for vitamin B_{12} is the classical microbiological assay using Lactobacillus. The technique appears to work well with raw commodities but not for processed foods that contain microbial growth inhibitors. The recently introduced protein-binding assays have been shown to respond to B_{12} isomers, which have no vitamin activity. Data on the correct vitamin B_{12} content of foods are therefore available for only a few foods, but sensitivity analysis will probably show that better, more complete analyses are only necessary for a few other foods.

Vitamin C. Both ascorbic acid and dehydroascorbic acid have vitamin C activity. There are several acceptable methods for measuring both forms. These appear to be adequate for assaying vitamin C in fresh products. Vitamin C is very labile to air oxidation, and the use of improper sample preparation can lead to an underestimation of the vitamin C content of fresh products.

In the case of processed foods, the situation is more difficult. Almost all the methods that measure the two forms of vitamin C also detect isoascorbic acid, and because isoascorbic acid is commonly used as an antioxidant in the food-processing industry, but has no vitamin C activity in humans, assays for the vitamin C content of processed foods have the potential for overestimating the vitamin C content.

Folacin. The class of chemical compounds named folacin consists of a complex mixture of chemical isomers with various oxidation states and different numbers of glutamate residues. There is no single chemical, biochemical, or microbiological assay that will accurately measure all the forms of this nutrient so they can be related to folacin activity in humans. Furthermore, the subcommittee does not know of any acceptable combination of techniques for measuring all the isomeric compounds with folacin activity.

The standard assay is a microbiological one that has differential responses to different isomers. It is not known whether or not humans have the same response to the individual folacin isomers as does Lactobacillus casei; however, there is no reason to assume that they do. It is known that there are a number of additional compounds that interfere with the existing assays or that alter the bioavailability of each folacin isomer. The interactions of these assay inhibitors and of compounds that alter the bioavailability are not well understood nor, apparently, have all the interfering compounds been identified.

An accurate, sensitive chemical assay for all the folacin isomers is needed to permit the resolution of the complex problems associated with assaying the folacin content of foods. Given the difficulties with assays of the folacin isomers, the data on the folacin content of food items do not appear to be reliable and the subcommittee does not believe that accurate estimates of the dietary intake of folacin can be obtained from the current food composition data bases.

IMPACT OF SYSTEMATIC BIAS

The preceding discussion has suggested that sources of random variation in either the food intake estimate or the food composition data affect confidence in the estimates of the prevalence of inadequate intake. For food intake data, the standard error of the composition data for individual foods may result in a relatively small under- or overestimation of prevalence. The models do not include systematic bias, such as that derived from consistent under- or overestimation of either total nutrient intake or the nutrient content of foods. The following paragraphs address the impact of that type of effect.

As noted, there are no valid estimates of the magnitude (if any) of bias in estimates of food intake from the NFCS data. The subcommittee emphasizes the need to determine if there is such a bias and if so, its extent so that the methods of estimation can be improved. An analagous situation holds for food composition data. In one study, Wolf (1981) estimated nutrient intakes from food records, from the 1963 USDA food composition data base (USDA, 1963), and from direct chemical analysis (see Table 7-1).

The analyses suggest that there was a definite bias toward overestimation of true iron intake. The low regression slope and correlation coefficient suggest that the bias may apply to only some classes of foods rather than to all foods. That is, there may have been a methodological error in the food composition table for some classes of foods.

USDA's food composition tables have been revised since those used by Wolf (1981). Major changes were made in the iron data for some classes of foods. At the request of the subcommittee, Wolf and his colleagues have recalculated the data from the original study by using the new food composition tables.

Table 7-1 indicates that there was a systematic bias in the earlier food composition tables, a bias that has now been removed for iron. The comparison illustrates also that bias in composition data must be investigated separately for each nutrient in each food composition table instead of being regarded as generically applicable. Marr (1971) has presented descriptions of several comparisons of calculated and measured intake; the direction of bias is inconsistent across studies and across nutri-

TABLE 7-1. Comparison of Calculated and Measured Food Intakes Using Revised Food Composition Tables for 22 Subjects[a]

Nutrient	Estimated Nutrient Intake		Group Mean (mg/day	
	Regression Equation	Correlation (R square)	Calculated[b]	Measured[c]
Calcium	Y = 0.82X + 71	0.89	832	762
Iron				
original	Y = 0.49X + 4.3	0.25	12.8	10.6
recalculation	Y = 0.83X + 2.09	0.33	10.5	10.6
Zinc	Y = 0.68X + 3.5	0.43	7.4	8.6
Copper	Y = 0.15X + 0.88	0.02	0.89	1.01
Potassium	Y = 0.82X + 0.26	0.72	2,680	2,370
Sodium	Y = 0.35X + 2.2	0.19	2,800	3,190

[a]From Wolf, 1981.
[b]Self-administered intake record.
[c]Chemically measured content of duplicate meal.

ents. Depending on the study design, such comparisons may be affected by variation and bias either in the food composition table alone or in combination with the food intake record.

When interpreting the results of such studies, one must recognize that the composition of individual food items vary and that the food composition table, at best, presents the average composition of a class of foods. That is, one should not expect perfect agreement between calculated and measured composition for an item of food or for a diet. This effect is demonstrated in Appendix E. Moreover, the introduction of this variation in composition (or, if one wishes, random variation) into the estimate of food composition in comparison to the true composition of the foods consumed will affect the slope of regression analyses in which calculated and directly measured composition are compared. To some degree, the flat slope syndrome described above and in the nutrition literature (e.g., Marr, 1971) can be attributed to this type of effect. (A similar phenomenon will occur if, for example, 1-day intakes are compared with multiple day intakes: the intraindividual variations in the data will be different, and this may affect the regression slope while leaving group mean comparisons unaffected.)

Although there are no direct estimates of the magnitude of bias that may exist in computed nutrient intakes reported in recent NFCS or other large-scale survey data bases, it is possible to demonstrate the potential effect of such bias on estimates of the prevalence of inadequate intake. This is illustrated for protein in Table 7-2. Here the observed distribution of intakes has been systematically increased or decreased by

TABLE 7-2. Potential Impact of Systematic Bias in Either Food Composition Tables or Food Estimates on Estimates of the Prevalence of Inadequate Intakes[a]

Adjustment to Intake Distribution (Mock Systematic Bias in Intake Estimate)	Group Mean Intake (g/day)	Estimated Prevalence (%)	Bias in Estimate (%)
Original + 20 g	111.2	0.1	− 2.1
Original + 15 g	106.2	0.3	− 1.9
Original + 10 g	101.2	0.7	− 1.5
Original + 5 g	96.2	1.2	− 1.0
Original	91.2	2.2	0
Original − 5 g	86.2	3.6	+ 1.4
Original − 10 g	81.2	5.6	+ 3.4
Original − 15 g	76.2	8.4	+ 6.2
Original − 20 g	71.2	12.3	+10.1

[a]Data from 1977-1978 NFCS for protein intake by adult males.

adding a constant amount of protein to each intake. This process shifts the total intake distribution upward or downward but does not change the shape of the distribution.

The magnitude of the effect on estimates of the prevalence of inadequate intake will depend on the relative positions of the distributions of intake and of requirement. Nevertheless, it is readily apparent that for any such estimate of adequacy, systematic bias in either food intake estimates or food composition data will result in erroneous estimates of prevalence. This effect is not specific to the probability approach. It would also occur if fixed cutoff points had been used.

8

Modeling of Sources of Variability and Biases

As discussed in the previous chapter, a number of errors and biases can arise when estimating the distribution of nutrient intake in a population. The estimated prevalence is derived directly from the estimated distribution of nutrient intake, as described by the probability approach. Therefore, errors and biases in the estimation of intake distribution will carry over to the estimation of prevalence. Identifying the different sources of error will enable us to assess the impact of these errors on the estimate of prevalence.

Some of the errors will be due to random sampling variation. The magnitude of these errors can be determined directly from the data, and their impact on prevalence estimates can be determined with statistical theory. Other sources of bias cannot be determined directly. It is, however, important to consider their impact on prevalence estimates. Once identified, indirect evidence or judgments can serve as a basis for estimating the magnitude of error, and sensitivity analysis can be used to determine how these errors may affect estimates of prevalence.

The first step in the Nationwide Food Consumption Survey (NFCS) is to select the respondents. Information on the previous day is elicited by interview. For the day of the interview and the following day, foods are recorded by respondents at the time of consumption. Foods are then assigned to categories for coding; the coded foods are converted to nutrients by multiplying the amount of food eaten by the nutrient content per 100 g. The nutrient content information is obtained from reference data on food composition, which are maintained and updated periodically by the U.S. Department of Agriculture (USDA).

In the following sections, the sources of error and bias are broken down according to random sampling errors, errors in reporting food intake, and errors in the food composition tables.

VARIABILITY DUE TO SAMPLING OF RESPONDENTS

In this discussion, errors in selecting respondents are presumed to arise randomly from an unclustered, unstratified random probability sample of the population. In this case, the prevalence estimate, p, has a standard error of $[p(1 - p)/N]^{1/2}$, where N is the size of the sample. These are presented in Table 8-1 and compared to the increases in standard errors when random variability in food intakes and food nutrient compositions are also taken into account. The proportional increases are relatively small and would be even smaller if one were to use the standard errors of the NFCS, which are slightly higher due to clustering.

RANDOM VARIABILITY IN FOODS CONSUMED

When sampling a population at random, many people are sampled for several days, and the amount of food eaten is classified according to many different food items or categories. The following system of notation will be used to examine the random variability: Different individuals will be denoted by the index i, different days by the index j, and different food items by the index k. For example, let A_{ijk} denote the amount of food eaten by the ith individual on the jth day of the kth food item category. When a random components model is used to model the errors resulting from a random sample, $A_{ijk} = \mu_k + I_{ik} + D_{ijk}$, where μ_k is the population mean amount of the kth food item eaten in one day and I_{ik} is the difference between the average amount of the kth food item eaten by individual i and the population mean. I_{ik} can be thought of as a random variable with values varying across a population centered at zero, i.e., $I_{ijk} = 0$ and variance is equal to $\sigma^2(I_k)$. The value $\sigma^2(I_k)$ is called the interindividual variability for that food. The term D_{ijk} refers to the difference in the amount of the kth food eaten on the jth day for the individual i and the average amount eaten by the individual i. The values D_{ijk} are also considered to be random variables varying across days for the same individual with mean zero and variance $\sigma^2(D_k)$. This is called the intraindividual variation for that food.

TABLE 8-1. The Mean and Standard Errors of Proportion with Inadequate Intake Resulting from Errors in Food Composition Tables for Different Nutrients for Males and Females. Contrasted to Estimates Obtained with the Delta Method when Table Errors Were Not Considered.

Nutrient	Error in Estimate	Proportion with Inadequate Intake, % (mean + standard error)	
		Male	Female
Protein	Delta[a]	1.2 + 0.19	7.2 + 0.52
	FCT[b]	1.2 + 0.32	7.2 + 1.1
Iron	Delta	2.7 + 0.31	NA[c]
	FCT	3.1 + 2.2	NA
Vitamin C	Delta	43.0 + 1.16	55.4 + 0.99
	FCT	43.0 + 1.55	55.4 + 1.13
Vitamin A	Delta	59.4 + 1.27	59.8 + 1.03
	FCT	59.5 + 2.18	59.7 + 1.89
Thiamin (mg/day)	Delta	32.2 + 1.04	NA
	FCT	32.2 + 5.85	NA
Thiamin (kcal/day)	Delta	2.6 + 0.36	NA
	FCT	3.4 + 2.49	NA
Vitamin C (minimum requirements)	Delta	0.25 + 0.06	1.13 + 0.16
	FCT	0.29 + 0.17	1.18 + 0.47

[a]Delta denotes error in estimates from variation in survey as obtained using the delta method (Bickel and Doksum, 1977) and includes sampling and reporting error only.

[b]FCT denotes error in estimate resulting from food composition tables, and includes sampling and reporting error.

[c]NA = Data were not available to the subcommittee.

Not all errors and biases will arise from random sampling. Some derive from the methods used in determining the amount of nutrient that a person consumes each day. Errors in reporting of foods eaten also require attention.

Previously, the amount of food consumed in one day was denoted by A_{ijk}. The actual amount of food reported by the subject will be denoted by $A^*_{ijk} = A_{ijk} + R\mu_k + RI_{ik} + RR_{ijk} + RB_k$. RR_{ijk} denotes the random error within an individual in reporting foods. The quantity is assumed to vary at random from day to day, and is centered at zero for each individual with variance equal to $\sigma^2(RR_k)$.

Some people may consistently overreport or underreport certain foods. The average of this consistent over- or underreporting of the kth food type across a population will be denoted by RB_k, and the ith individual's over- or underreporting will be denoted by RI_{ik}. The variable RI_{ik} varies across individuals in a population and is centered at zero with a variance of $\sigma^2(RI_k)$. The value of RB_k is assumed to be a constant.

Random error in food reporting enters into intraindividual variation. Because the adjustment of the intake distribution described in Chapter 4 separates interindividual variation from intraindividual variation, this type of intraindividual reporting error will have no effect on the estimation of prevalence.

Consistent under- or overreporting of food intake will be part of the interindividual variation and will not be removed in the adjustment of intake data. Thus, it can affect the estimate of prevalence. The value $\sigma^2(RI)$, if it exists, would contribute to the true interindividual variation and, hence, would artificially inflate the spread of the actual intake distribution. The standard deviation for the intake distribution, which should be σCI, will be estimated by $[\sigma^2(I) + \sigma^2(RI)]^{1/2}$. Unless $\sigma^2(RI)$ is substantially large, this will have little effect on the prevalence estimates. For example, the coefficient of variation of the interindividual variation for many of the nutrients range from 30% to 50% (see Appendix A). If the over- and underreporting errors are symmetrical but on the order of 10% so that $\sigma^2(RI)$ has a CV of about 10%, then this would inflate the CV from 30% to 32% or from 50% to 51%. Similarly, if the reporting errors are on the order of $\pm$ 20%, then this would inflate the CV from 30% to 36% or from 50% to 54%.

This is not true, however, if the over- and underreporting is not symmetrical, that is, if there is an overall systematic bias in reporting for the entire population or when the bias term RB is not equal to zero. This, however, is not true of the bias term RB_k. Sensitivity analyses have shown that changes in the mean could have a substantial effect on the estimate of prevalence. Hence, systematic over- or underreporting of certain foods by a population must be taken very seriously.

VARIABILITY IN FOOD COMPOSITION DATA

Using statistical notation, one can summarize the errors and biases that may occur in the compilation of food composition tables. When the amount of nutrient per 100 g of a food item is to be measured, the analysis is performed on a theoretically representative sample of the food. Although the food composition tables (USDA, 1976-1984) give a single number representing the mean nutrient content per 100 g of the food item, the importance of the distribution of nutrients per food item must be recognized.

To examine the impact of possible errors in these data, let us denote F_k as the true mean nutrient content for the distribution of the kth food item. Let FR_{ijk} denote the difference between the mean nutrient content F_k and the actual amount of nutrient in the kth food eaten by the ith individual on the jth day. The variable FR_{ijk} is assumed to be randomly distributed with a mean of zero and a variance of $\sigma^2 FR_k$. The variance represents the true variability of nutrient content that is found within a population of certain types of food items. It is assumed that the foods eaten from day to day are random samples from this distribution.

If people do not randomly select their foods from a group of specific food items but, rather, systematically and regularly select specific items (e.g., a certain brand of fortified cereal rather than samples of many kinds of cereals), then bias will be introduced. This bias will be denoted by the term FB_{ik}--the difference between the average amount of nutrient that the ith individual eats and the population mean F_k. It can be assumed that the variable FB_{ik} varies from individual to individual and is centered at zero with a variance of $\sigma^2 FB_k$.

Finally, C_k will be used to denote the difference between the true mean nutrient content F_k and the content as estimated from the food composition tables. The value C_k includes many components of error, such as laboratory error, sampling error, and biases, in relation to foods for laboratory analysis. Estimates of the nutrient content of foods are obtained by averaging the content of food samples.

Ideally, the recorded nutrient intake equals the true amount of food eaten multiplied by the true nutrient content of the foods and summed over all food items. Hence, the <u>actual</u> amount of nutrient intake for the ith individual on the jth day could be expressed as

$$N_{ij} = \Sigma(\mu_k + I_{ik} + D_{ijk})(F_k + FB_{ik} + FR_{ijk}).$$

The measured nutrient content is the amount of food reported, multiplied by the nutrient content of each food as given in the food tables and summed over all food items. The following expression describes the measured nutrient content of the ith individual on the jth day:

$$N_{ij}^* = \sum_k(\mu_k + I_{ik} + D_{ijk} + RI_{ik} + RR_{ijk})(F_k + C_k).$$

The difference between the true nutrient intake and the measured nutrient intake is:

$$N_{ij}^* - N_{ij} = \sum_k(FB_{ik} + FR_{ijk} - C_k)(\mu_k + I_{ik} + D_{ijk})$$
$$- \sum_k C_k(RB_k + RI_{ik} + RR_{ijk}).$$

When there is no systematic bias in the reporting of foods, the following conditions apply: RB_k and RI_{ik} are both equal to zero, and there is no systematic bias in the ways individuals select particular kinds of food, i.e., FB_{ijk} is equal to zero. Under these constraints, where the only errors are random,

$$N_{ij}^* = N_{ij} + \sum_k FR_{ijk}(\mu_k + I_{ik} + D_{ijk}) + \sum_k C_k(RR_{ijk})$$
$$+ D_{ijk} + \Sigma C_k \mu_k + \sum_k C_k I_{ik}.$$

This can be written as

$$N_{ij}^* = N_{ij} + X + Y_i + Z_{ij},$$

where $X = \Sigma C_k \mu_k$, $Y_i = \sum_k C_k I_{ik}$, and $Z_{ij} = \sum_k FR_{ijk}(\mu_k + I_{ijk}) + D_{ijk} + \Sigma C_k (RR_{ijk} + D_{ijk})$.

We now turn to estimating the effects of these errors on prevalence estimates.

EFFECT OF RANDOM STATISTICAL ERROR ON ESTIMATION OF PREVALENCE

The amount of nutrient intake is estimated for each person on each day of the survey from information about food consumed obtained in the survey together with the food composition tables. As described in detail in Appendix C, two approaches for estimating prevalence have been suggested: the parametric approach, which assumes that the distribution of nutrient intake, or some transformation of the data, is normal, and the nonparametric approach, which does not make this assumption.

The nonparametric approach would probably be the preferred method for estimating prevalence; however, the statistical methods used are much more difficult to model than those in the parametric approach. For this reason, the parametric approach is used in this chapter to generate an approximate measure of the degree of variability in the estimate of prevelance. Where the estimates of prevalence calculated in the two approaches differ, this should only be slight; however, in such a case the estimate obtained with the nonparametric approach is the one of choice.

As indicated in Appendix C, prevalence estimates based on the parametric approach are derived from the population means of interindividual variation of nutrient intake, which are obtained from an analysis of variance (ANOVA) of the nutrient data. If the nutrient content recorded for each subject on each day of observation is exactly correct, then the only error in estimating prevalence would be statistical fluctuation resulting from random sampling. The magnitude of this statistical fluctuation will be measured by the standard error of the estimate.

The formulas and theory necessary to find the standard error of the prevalence estimate are given in Appendix C.

The assumption was made that the distribution of actual intakes was log-normal.

When a log-normal distribution is assumed, this method may not be appropriate and a larger class of transformations should be considered (Box and Cox, 1964). However, the major purpose of this exercise is to get some sense of the degree of statistical variation in the estimation procedure. For this purpose, the log-normal assumption will be adequate. To obtain 95% confidence intervals, the estimate ± 2 standard errors could be used.

As was noted previously, the amount of nutrient recorded does not exactly reflect the amount of nutrient ingested. In fact, even when there is no systematic bias in the reporting or choices of foods eaten,

$$N_{ij}^* = N_{ij} + X + Y_i + Z_{ij},$$

where N_{ij}^* is the amount of nutrient <u>reported</u> from the ith individual on day j and N_{ij} is the <u>actual</u> amount of nutrient for the ith individual on day j.

The component Z_{ij} is incorporated as part of the day-to-day variability and will be taken out by the analysis of variance. Hence, Z_{ij} will not have any effect on the estimate of standard error of proportion with inadequate intake.

In the probability approach, an analysis of variance of the true N_{ij} should be used to estimate the population mean of the nutrient and interindividual variation. These estimates are then used to estimate the proportion with inadequate intake. In actuality, however, the analysis of variance is made on the N_{ij}^*. Hence, the population mean that is being estimated is the true population mean $\Sigma F_k \mu_k$ plus the value X, which is a realization of the error terms coming from the food tables. Also, the interindividual variation that is being estimated is equal to the true interindividual variation plus the variance of Y_i.

Y_i has a minimal effect on the estimate of interindividual variation and almost no effect on the estimate of proportion with inadequate intake. Therefore, we shall only consider the effect of error term X on the estimate of proportion with inadequate intake.

The proportion of the population with inadequate intake, say P, is a function of the population mean and inter-individual variation σ_I^2. That is, $P = S(\mu \sigma_I^2)$. As mentioned previously, we are estimating $P^* = S(\mu + X\sigma_I^2)$, where $X = \Sigma C_k \mu_k$ can be thought of as a random variable with a mean of zero and a variance equal to $\sum_k \mu_k^2 \text{Var} C_k$.

To derive some sense of how much P* could be expected to vary from P, a sensitivity analysis was performed in the following manner. First, it was necessary to assign an approximate value for the variance, which will be denoted by $\sigma_B^2 = \sum_k \mu_k^2 \text{Var} C_k$. (More will be said about this later.) Random values X_1, X_2, ..., X_{500} are generated from the distribution of X, assumed to be normally distributed with mean zero and variance σ_B^2. Values of $P_i^* = S(\mu + X_i, \sigma_I^2)$ were computed as were their mean and standard deviation. The values of μ and σ_I^2 are estimates obtained from the original analysis of variance. Although the exercise will not produce precise estimates of the standard error resulting from food composition tables, it can be used to assess the impact of errors in food tables on the estimates of the prevalence of inadequate intake.

To estimate σ_B^2, the standard error in the mean nutrient composition was obtained for a typical diet. The most recent set of reference tables on food composition that have been published by the USDA (1976-1984) provide some information about the number of samples analyzed and the standard error of the mean for some foods. Using method-ology similar to that described in Appendix E (using standard error instead of standard deviation), the sub-committee obtained a rough approximation of the standard error in the mean nutrient consumed in a sample diet as a result of random sampling of foods from the food composition table.

In all cases, the estimation errors relating to the errors in food composition tables are larger than errors resulting from the survey data. The effect of the errors in the food table on estimates of prevalence cannot be diminished by larger surveys. Improvement can be made only with more accurate food tables.

IMPACT OF RANDOM UNDER- AND OVERREPORTING

A number of the dietary methodology studies reported in Chapter 6 suggest that there may be under- and over-reporting of intake. This is to be distinguished from

systematic misreporting by a population or population group
(see Chapter 7). If the random element relates to
individual reporting from day to day, the effect will be
removed during the process of adjusting the distribution to
remove the impact of day-to-day variation. However, if some
people systematically underreport while others systematically overreport, the between-individual variance will be
incorporated in the estimate of the distribution of usual
intake. This effect can be expected to have an impact on
estimates of the prevalence of inadequate intake. The
subcommittee used a series of simulations to examine the
nature and magnitude of the impact.

To provide some perspective on the potential magnitude of
interindividual random under- and overreporting, Table 8-2
portrays, using simulation techniques, the effects that might
be seen in population data if there is bias in reporting by
an individual. A comparison of observed and reported intakes
for single meals is discussed by Schnakenberg et al. (1981).
In their data, there was an apparent overall bias toward
underestimation. Of more importance for the present purpose,

TABLE 8-2. Magnitude of Expected Effect of Random Under-
and Overreporting in Population Data[a]

Coefficient of Variation (% of Mean)	Distribution of Deviations Between Recorded and True Intake (% of Subjects Exhibiting Deviation)					
	30%	25%	20%	15%	10%	5%
5	2.7	3.4	4.2	5.2	6.4	8.2
10	5.3	6.7	8.4	10.4	12.8	16.5
15	7.8	10.1	12.6	15.5	19.2	24.7
20	10.5	13.5	16.8	20.7	25.6	32.9
25	13.1	16.8	21.0	25.9	32.0	41.1
30	15.8	20.2	25.2	31.1	38.4	49.4

[a]The body of the table displays the magnitude of the
deviation between recorded intake and a measure of true
intake that would be expected in the proportion of subjects specified in the column. Deviations of the magnitude shown or greater would be expected. Assumes a
Gaussian distribution for this simulation.

the standard deviation of misreporting expressed as a proportion of observed intake was 28% of the mean score (32%) for protein. This demonstrates the magnitude of under- and overreporting of single meals. Unless there is evidence that each person is consistent in his or her misreporting, the measured variance must include an unmeasured proportion of intraindividual variation. That is, the CV of 30% overestimates the error that would be expected in estimates of the distribution of usual intake (i.e., intake across multiple meals per day and many days). Many other studies cited in Chapter 7, in which one dietary methodology was compared with another in reporting under- and overestimation, fail to take into account the impact of differences in the number of days of observation. Thus, the literature does not provide a direct estimate of the magnitude of under- and overreporting that might be expected in data sets adjusted to remove day-to-day variability of intake. The report of Schnakenberg et al. (1981) indicates that a realistic worst-case situation would be a CV of 20% for misreporting the estimate of usual intake distributions.

The potential effects of random interindividual misreporting on estimates of the prevalence of inadequate intakes can be simulated as shown in Table 8-3. The adjusted distributions of usual intake for protein and for vitamin C (Appendix A) were further adjusted to incorporate or to remove the effect of a component of random variation. This was done by using ratios of standard deviations of the derived distribution of usual intakes. The standard deviations adjusted to add or remove a variance component are used in the same manner as reported in Appendix A, except that the distributions were not normalized first. The approach preserves the skew of the distribution of usual intakes. The probability approach was then used to derive estimates of the apparent prevalence of inadequate intakes.

From these simulations it can be seen that random interindividual under- and overreporting of intake can affect the prevalence estimate. Consideration of the underlying theory indicates that the magnitude of the effect will depend on the magnitude of the variance of this component in relation to the true interindividual variation as well as on the means of the intake and requirement distributions. In the case of protein, with the estimated variation of usual intakes (see Appendix

TABLE 8-3.   Potential Impact of Random Interindividual Misreporting of Intake on the Estimate of Prevalence of Inadequate Intakes in Adult Males

CV[a] of Random Error (%)	Impact of Addition of Error Term (%)[b]		Impact of Removing Error Term (%)	
	Protein	Vitamin C	Protein	Vitamin C
0	2.1	41.0	2.1	41.0
5	2.3	41.1	2.0	41.0
10	2.8	41.3	1.5	40.8
15	3.7	41.6	0.8	40.4
20	4.9	42.1	0.2	39.8
25	6.5	42.6	0	39.1
30	8.3	43.1	c	38.0

[a]CV = coefficient of variation.
[b]Values are the apparent prevalences of inadequate intake computed by the probability approach. Mean requirement of protein taken as 43 g/day and mean requirement of vitamin C taken as 46.2 mg/day. CV of requirement taken as 15% of the mean.
[c]Cannot be computed. In this case the error term would be equal to or greater than the estimated interindividual variation--an impossible situation.

A) much smaller than that of vitamin C, the impact of adding or removing a component of variance would be much greater. The requirement and intake distributions for protein are also much more widely separated than in the case of vitamin C, which would accentuate the effect. Protein then can be used as a worst-case scenario.

Table 8-3 also gives the potential effects of removing an independent variance component. In the NFCS data set, the potential impact of removing a component of variance is of particular interest. Removing the variance component permits examination of any bias that might be present in the estimate of prevalence because of random under- and overreporting present in the original data set, whereas addition of variance would arise only if there was evidence of a negative correlation between intake and overestimation. In this case, the correlation itself would have to be considered.

The 20% estimate of the CV used here would be a generous estimate of the possible variation attributable to this source, and the analysis shown in Table 8-3 suggests that the impact, although real, would not be serious. The prevalence estimate for protein might fall from 2.1% to 0.2%, both of which would be considered very low prevalences. This analysis has used a worst-case scenario with a high error term and a prevalence of inadequate intake that falls in the tail of the intake distribution. In contrast, the prevalence estimate for vitamin C might change from 41.0% to 39.8%--an operationally undetectable change. Only if it could be argued that the random error greatly exceeds the real variation, after day-to-day variability had been factored out, would the magnitude of the error be totally unacceptable for the purpose of survey data interpretation. Again the subcommittee emphasizes that this phenomenon is quite different from systematic under- or overreporting across individuals. That effect is discussed as bias in the estimate of intake earlier in this chapter.

9

Conclusions and Recommendations

In keeping with its mandate, the subcommittee's main suggestion is the adoption of a new approach to the interpretation of dietary intake data that are collected in large surveys such as the Nationwide Food Consumption Survey (NFCS). The subcommittee has also recommended changes in the design of these surveys to facilitate or improve the reliability of interpretations of nutritional adequacy and to improve the data bases, thereby facilitating application of the recommended approach. Some of these recommendations are applicable immediately, even retrospectively, to existing data from surveys, whereas others could be implemented in the next NFCS survey. Still others relate to longer range activities and research programs sponsored by U.S. Department of Agriculture (USDA) and other agencies. Although the subcommittee recognizes that recommendations related to longer term activities will require more time for implementation, it urges that immediate steps be taken toward their adoption in view of their importance.

ANALYSIS OF DIETARY ADEQUACY

The subcommittee concluded that many disadvantages and erroneous interpretations are associated with the application of fixed cutoff points, i.e., the Recommended Dietary Allowances (RDAs) or percentages of them, as criteria for the interpretation of observed nutrient intake and that the use of fixed cutoff points may lead to erroneous estimates of the prevalence of inadequate intake.

• The subcommittee recommends that a probability approach to the interpretation of computed nutrient intake be developed and adopted, where feasible. This approach would lead to estimates of the prevalence of inadequate intake among individuals in the total population and in population subgroups. This approach is not necessary for nutrients consumed in excess of the RDA by almost all members of the population, for whom adequacy of nutrient intake can be assumed.

The subcommittee recognizes that nutritional assessments based on multiple levels of adequacy are important to government agencies and others for use in planning various nutrition programs and in reaching a better understanding of the nutritional needs of the U.S. population. With a multilevel approach, for example, one might look at the intake levels deemed inadequate to prevent clinical manifestations of deficiency, to maintain the functional integrity of metabolic systems, or to maintain high tissue concentrations of nutrients if that level is continued for a long period. Each of these levels is different. Although the subcommittee did not propose a particular set of criteria for this multilevel approach, it concluded that a multilevel assessment of expected dietary adequacy in the U.S. population will provide a more useful picture of nutritional adequacy for planners.

• The subcommittee further recommends the development of multiple criteria for nutritional adequacy and estimates of intake required to maintain the various levels of adequacy.

To implement the probability approach, it is necessary to bring together information about the distribution of nutrient requirements among similar persons (e.g., young adult males, young adult females, children of specified ages). This information about the distribution of nutrient requirements is not always presented in directly applicable form in the Recommended Dietary Allowances (NRC, 1980) or in other reports, although it might be derived from the studies that are reviewed in the text of such reports. Sensitivity analyses have shown that estimates of the average requirement and some idea about the symmetry of the distribution are more important than a precise estimate of the variability. To implement the first recommendation given above, such information must be reviewed and judgments must be made about the distributions.

• The subcommittee recommends that working descriptions of the distributions of nutrient requirements be developed

and improved. Such descriptions should place major
emphasis on deriving estimates of, or judgments about,
both the central tendency of the distribution and the
symmetry of the distribution. Although precise knowledge
of the characteristics of the distribution is desirable,
it is not essential; estimates of the range can be used.

The probability approach proposed in this report pre-
cludes the classification of individuals as having adequate or inadequate diets. In addition, it would be very
difficult, if not impossible, to estimate the proportion of
populations with multiple dietary inadequacies. For subgroups of the population, however, it is possible to estimate the prevalence of deficiency for separate nutrients.
Thus the existence of multiple inadequacies in a population
group and possibly in different people can be estimated,
even though this is not possible for individuals.

• The subcommittee recommends that multiple dietary
inadequacies be assessed from NFCS data only for populations and subpopulations--not for individuals.

The probability approach cannot be applied to the interpretation of observed energy intake, even if perfectly measured, because the intake and requirements are highly correlated in well-fed populations such as that of the United
States.

• The subcommittee recommends that the probability
approach not be applied to the interpretation of observed
energy intake. In well-fed populations, energy status as
judged by stores must be assessed by anthropometry. Energy
intake might be viewed as a potential measure of the implied
distribution of physical activity in the total population
and in population subgroups.

The subcommittee concluded that for some nutrients, it
is inappropriate to base inadequate intake estimates on
dietary information. Major environmental variables that
influence requirement (e.g., the importance of sunlight
exposure in the determination of vitamin D requirements)
have not yet been assessed for all nutrients. Moreoever,
information about requirements is often fragmentary (e.g.,
for calcium) and data on current food composition may be
inadequate (e.g., for folate). For these nutrients, it is
nevertheless appropriate to derive descriptive information
about observed intake and to make comparisons among subpopu-

lations, even though the assessment cannot be made as accurately as for the majority of nutrients.

● The subcommittee recommends that prevalence estimates of inadequate intakes be attempted for nutrients only when acceptable information about requirements and adequate food composition data are available.

● When no probability assessment can be made for a nutrient, the subcommittee recommends the descriptive presentation of the mean, variance, and percentile distributions.

With the probability approach described in this report, one can estimate the absolute prevalence of inadequate dietary intakes, defined as intakes that will not maintain appropriate biochemical stores or functions. Many uses of the NFCS do not require such absolute prevalence estimates. In particular, differences between population groups can be determined with other statistically more powerful methods.

● The subcommittee recommends that the probability approach not be used to generate prevalence estimates for statistical testing of comparisons between or among subpopulations for which statistically more powerful methods exist.

In the judgment of the subcommittee, all the above recommendations can be applied immediately. The probability approach can be investigated, developed, and implemented with several existing survey data bases.

STUDY DESIGN

The interpretation of the probability approach and its application to the assessment of observed nutrient intake involves several important statistical considerations. These considerations should help to determine the design of data collection, the methods of analysis, and the interpretation.

A major requirement for the application of the probability approach, or any other approach used to interpret the distribution of observed intakes, is the use of statistical procedures that take into account the effect of day-to-day variation in nutrient intake within the individual. The subcommittee addressed this matter and outlined procedures for implementation. Absolute prerequisites for these procedures are repeated observations on individual daily intake. There must be sufficient numbers of replications for population subgroups as well as for the population as a whole. The precise number of replications needed should be considered when designing the survey. Moreover, there appears to be an increase in statistical power if the replicated 1-day intake estimates are obtained by the same method and on independent rather than on adjacent days. It is important also to sample days of the week in the design and to include questions on dietary supplements as well as on food intake.

Considering these survey design requirements and the previously identified need for statistical services in connection with analysis and interpretation, the subcommittee makes the following recommendations:

● The scope of the statistical services that are integral to the design, analysis, and interpretation of the NFCS should be reinforced and expanded.

● During the planning of future surveys, the following aspects of the design should be considered: (1) the number and distribution of replicate intakes required for statistically reliable adjustments of the distribution of observed intakes to estimate the distribution of usual intakes for the population and subgroups, (2) the wisdom and feasibility of modifying data collection to include a single method for use over all days of observation rather than the two systems presently used to collect dietary information, and (3) the need and feasibility of sampling on independent rather than on consecutive days.

● Investigations of dietary methodology should continue to be presented and published in order to obtain additional information on such matters as (1) the association between intake estimates made on the first days of observation and those made on subsequent days (correlation of intake across days) and hence the relative importance of sampling on independent days and (2) sampling, respondent, or interviewer biases that may affect the reliability of population intake estimates and hence methodological approaches that might avoid or minimize any biases that do exist. The characteristics of respondents likely to have biases in reported intake data should be identified, and the direction, and where possible the magnitude, of the biases should be estimated. Priorities for methodological research of this kind for the NFCS should include statistical considerations pertinent to the planning of survey design, data analysis, and data interpretation.

Because the assessment of inadequate (or excessive) nutrient intake is not the only important use for NFCS data, the subcommittee concluded that data requirements for other applications may differ from those identified in the present report or implied by the recommendations contained herein. Thus, it will be necessary to consider all intended purposes of the survey during the design phase.

● The subcommittee recommends that the USDA review the important uses of the data to ensure that the survey design is adequate for an appropriate balance among these uses.

SENSITIVITY ANALYSIS

Although the subcommittee did not arrange the recommendations in any order of priority, the report does show some of the approaches that might be used to derive a priority ranking. For example, it is possible to test the effect of including food composition errors in estimates of the prevalence of inadequate intake. (See examples presented in this report for testing the sensitivity of the prediction to variability of requirement, to errors in estimates of nutrient intake, and to variability of food composition.) The relative effect of various sources of error on estimations of the prevalence of inadequate or excessive intakes can be identified. To the extent that these effects of error differ between nutrients, they can be used to establish priority ranking for nutrients. In addition to these considerations, the relative cost of reducing an identified source of error should be considered in judgments about priorities for data improvements.

The following recommendations, then, are not presented in any order of priority, although these actions should be implemented to the extent that resources permit.

IMPROVEMENT OF THE FOOD COMPOSITION DATA BASE

The discussions in Chapters 7 and 8 and in Appendices C
and E have illustrated that bias and variation in food composition data can have a significant impact on prevalence
estimates. The subcommittee recommends that the USDA
recognize the importance of the food composition data to
the accuracy of the such estimates and that it implement
the recommendations in this chapter.

The subcommittee recognizes the need to improve the data
base on almost all nutrients in some foods and on some
nutrients in almost all foods. It also recognizes that such
improvements may have limited importance for public policy
purposes either because there is little or no public health
concern about the nutrient and, hence, limited reason to
improve precision of estimates or because the missing or
unreliable data refer to foods that make a minor contribution to intakes and, hence, whose errors have minimal
impact on the estimate of prevalence of inadequate intakes.
The subcommittee has not attempted to judge or assess the
relative priorities for improving the data base. Rather, it
has chosen to recommend areas where improvements could be
made. Before these recommendations are assigned relative
priorities, sensitivity analyses of the type presented in
this report should be conducted to establish whether or not
improvement of the data base would have practical
significance.

The subcommittee was asked to discuss four nutrients for
which there are inadequate methodologies. Of these, folacin, the carotenoids, and vitamin C may be of present or
future public health significance in the United States.
Existing methodologies are also inadequate for Vitamin B_{12}.

● Thus the subcommittee recommends that the USDA provide the necessary resources for developing an adequate
methodology for assaying folacin, the carotenoids, vitamin
B_{12}, and vitamin C in foods if justified by their public
health significance and by sensitivity analysis.

For the other nutrients listed in the charge to the
subcommittee for which there are adequate analytical methodologies, there are a number of foods for which there either
are no data or only imputed data. For some foods, nutrient
values are determined by adding the individual ingredients
listed in the formulation rather than by direct analysis.

• Given the potential impact of imputed data on the prevalence estimates, the subcommittee recommends that the USDA impute values in the food composition data bases so that no zero values are substituted by default for missing values.

• The USDA should differentiate between imputed values and values that are calculated or determined by laboratory analyses in food composition data bases and clearly identify calculated and imputed values so that users can readily differentiate among these values when interpreting the prevalence estimates.

The subcommittee believes that priorities for the acquisition of new analytical data should be based on the contribution of the food to the nutrient intake of the population.

• Therefore the subcommittee recommends that the USDA perform sensitivity analyses on the imputed values of all foods for which data on key nutrients are missing to determine the probable impact of these foods on the total nutrient intake in the populations of interest.

When the results of the sensitivity analyses are known, the subcommittee recommends that the USDA perform the following functions:

• It should collect analytical data for foods containing nutrients shown by sensitivity analyses to have the greatest impact on prevalence estimates.

• It should ensure that the foods sampled represent the total foods consumed in the United States. Where the range of nutrient composition for a currently classified food is wide, it should consider subdividing the existing classification into smaller groups with narrower ranges of composition. Such restructuring may be most appropriate for processed foods as was the case for breakfast cereals in the current data bases. Again, this decision should be preceded by sensitivity analysis.

• The USDA should also increase the number of assays for selected nutrients to decrease standard errors of the mean, where sensitivity analyses indicate that the precision of the prevalence estimates will be significantly improved.

The subcommittee believes that the usefulness of the dietary survey data bases can be improved. Toward this end, it recommends the following:

● The USDA should publish and document the algorithms and procedures used in the computation of the nutrient intakes and their variance, the means and the standard error of the means in food composition data bases, and the prevalence estimates and their variances.

● The USDA should publish the concentrations of the individual isomers of the nutrients in food composition data bases, tables, and dietary intake data tapes.

The subcommittee believes that the bioavailability of some nutrients may affect prevalence estimates. Thus the subcommittee recommends the following:

● The USDA should promote and support research that leads to an understanding of the major factors that influence the bioavailability of key nutrients and the development of algorithms for predicting the bioavailability of these nutrients in meals.

● When the understanding and algorithms have been developed, the agency should use sensitivity analysis to assess the impact of including bioavailability in the calculation of prevalence estimates. Further actions should be based on the outcome of these sensitivity analyses.

The subcommittee believes that public interest in the maintenance of optimal health will continue and that the food consumption surveys will be expected to provide more information on this aspect of diet and public health. Many of the dietary components believed to enhance or retard the development of diseases such as cancer and cardiovascular disease have not traditionally been listed in food composition tables. Thus it has not been possible to assess dietary intake of such compounds in the population through the food consumption surveys. The subcommittee believes that listing these compounds in the food composition tables would significantly enhance the ability of the USDA to respond to anticipated questions on the intake of food components by the U.S. public and will provide the U.S. population with much better information on the adequacy and safety of its diet. However, the analysis necessary to acquire this information could also be very costly. Thus the sub-committee recommends the following:

• The USDA should investigate the possibility of ex-panding the food composition data bases to include listings for all compounds in foods that are believed to affect human health so that the intake of these components can be assessed in future surveys.

• Where potential health benefit is likely, and the quality of the chemical analysis warrants, the USDA should analyze these components, many of which are not nutrients, and include them in the food composition data bases.

PREREQUISITES AND LIMITATIONS OF THE PROPOSED APPROACH

The subcommittee is aware that its report poses a number of questions regarding the immediate application of the pro-posed approach to the analysis of nutrient intake data. As indicated by the report of one member (see pp. 104-109), there was not complete agreement about the practicality of the approach. All members of the subcommittee are in agree-ment on the scientific validity of the proposed approach and on the nature of these unresolved issues relating to survey design and data base adequacy; however, opinion varied as to the probability of success in developing the information needed to apply the approach and the time that will be needed for the required research. The subcom-mittee's judgments are presented under four major areas: acceptable precision of estimates of the prevalence of inadequate intake, estimation of usual food intake, compu-tation of nutrient intake, and definition of nutrient requirements.

Acceptable Precision of the Estimates

Consideration of the use of estimates of the prevalence of inadequate intakes and of the overall implication of the proposed approach led the subcommittee to discuss the ac-ceptable level of accuracy for prevalence estimates. In Chapter 8, estimates of the confidence intervals for esti-mates of the prevalence of inadequate intake are presented. These take into account all recognized potential sources of bias in the prevalence estimate with the exception of systematic bias in reporting intake or misestimation of

mean requirement. In the considered judgment of members of
the subcommittee, errors even severalfold greater than
those estimated in Chapter 8 would be acceptable for policy
analyses. On this all members of the subcommittee agreed.
The areas of differing opinion within the subcommittee
concerned ideas about the magnitude of unmeasured errors.

Estimation of Usual Food Intake

The omission of homeless and institutionalized persons
from the sampling frame for the NFCS has already been
mentioned in Chapter 7. This omission will lead to systematic underrepresentation of the population at highest
risk of nutritional deficits, thereby biasing the results
of the study to some extent. The subcommittee has recommended further research to estimate the magnitude of this
bias and to reduce it. This appears to be amenable to satisfactory resolution through applied research and appropriate survey design, including collaboration with other
national surveys. Even though NFCS may continue to under-
sample or omit certain segments of the population, it may
be possible to gain information about these segments from
other surveys, thus complementing NFCS information without
necessitating a radical change in the NFCS design. Any
residual limitations of the design, and hence the need to
draw upon other information, should be made clear to users.

The subcommittee recognizes that subjects may vary in
the reliability with which they report food ingested.
There may be random under- and overreporting by one subject across days. A subject may consistently under- or
overreport, but this may be random between subjects. Or,
the entire group may systematically under- or overreport.
The nature and extent of these effects in the NFCS are not
known. In Chapter 7, the subcommittee considered the
potential impact of variations in reporting and concluded
that random variation in the reports of one subject would
have no impact on the prevalence estimate derived by the
proposed method. Random variation between subjects would
have an effect on the estimate. Within the plausible range
of magnitude of these effects, however, the bias introduced
in the prevalence estimate would be acceptable for policy
applications of the results. The subcommittee concluded
that a serious potential effect would derive from any
appreciable systematic under- or overreporting across the
entire population or subpopulation under study. In the

absence of specific information about the magnitude of this
phenomenon, if it exists in the NFCS, opinions about reliability of the prevalence estimates varied. For those
members who believed the problem to be large, there were
also differences of opinion about the feasibility of
improving the collection of data on dietary intake and
analytical procedures to minimize the impact on the prevalence estimates. There was unanimous agreement that the
USDA should continue its efforts to assess the magnitude of
reporting bias. If bias is found, the USDA should increase
its efforts to improve methods for collecting data on
reduction of bias in dietary intake data and analytical
methods to correct for known bias in derivations of the
prevalence estimate.

The subcommittee emphasizes that where other information
documents the existence of a nutritional problem in the
population, meaningful comparison of intakes between population groups can be made without use of the probability
approach.

Computation of Nutrient Intake

As was discussed in Chapter 7, error can also enter into
the estimates during the conversion of food intake data into
nutrient composition data. This process is dependent on the
sampling of foods for chemical analysis, the analytical
methods used, the coding categories used to describe foods
in the food composition data set, and the computation of
nutrient intake. The greatest potential for error in this
process is associated with the analytical methods selected
and the representativeness with which foods are sampled.
The subcommittee believes that the analytical methods for
vitamin C and folate and for the vitamin A carotenoids may
produce inaccurate data and that sensitivity analysis is
required to determine the extent of this effect on the
probable outcome of improved assays for these nutrients.
The results of these sensitivity analyses should indicate
whether it would be worthwhile to develop better analytical
methods to correct errors in the existing data. Improvements of this kind are feasible.

Error may also be introduced into the estimates during
the computation of nutrient intake. The subcommittee concluded that imputed values may be a source of such error
and calls for identification of imputed values in the data

sets on nutrient composition. The significance of the
impact of imputed values should also be determined through
sensitivity analysis. Selective assaying of foods shown by
the sensitivity analysis to be responsible for errors in
the final data could then be undertaken. Again the subcommittee believes that action can be taken to manage this
issue.

Members of the subcommittee agreed that variations in
the bioavailability of nutrients will produce errors in
estimations of the nutrient intake of a person. However,
across individuals, the effect may be no more important
than the random under- and overreporting across individuals, as considered earlier. Opinions varied as to the
present importance of the problem and the potential for
its solution. Nutrients for which errors are likely to
have the greatest impact are iron, zinc, and folate.

The subcommittee unanimously agreed that errors in the
computer algorithm for computations of any nutrients, to
the extent that they exist, would have an impact on the
estimates and that these can and should be corrected.

Definition of Nutrient Requirements

As was discussed in detail in Chapter 3, information on
the mean and approximate symmetry of the nutrient requirement is needed in order to apply the probability approach.
Analyses performed by the subcommittee and presented in
Chapter 5 show that differences in the standard deviation
and range of the distribution have a minimal effect on the
estimates as long as the distribution is symmetrical.
Therefore, imprecision in the description of the variance
of requirement was not a major issue. Lack of information
on mean nutrient requirement was a major concern for all
members of the subcommittee; however, views on the precision of the requisite estimates of mean nutrient requirement varied. Some members believed that reasonable estimates of mean requirement can be constructed immediately
for many nutrients across requisite age and sex groups and
that these estimates will provide a rational basis for
analysis. Others believe that more definitive and scientifically validated estimates are required. In the face of
these differing opinions on the level of specificity and
criteria of proof needed for mean requirement data, there
was a lack of agreement on the likelihood of developing
this information in the foreseeable future.

There was agreement in recommending that multiple levels of requirement, reflecting a series of states of nutriture, be developed and applied. These might relate, for example, to the prevention of scurvy on the one hand and to the maintenance of tissue stores of ascorbic acid on the other. There was recognition that ascorbic acid may have other effects, perhaps unrelated to its nutrient properties, such as anticarcinogenicity. Requirements to achieve this effect are not known. Other nutrients may require similar considerations. All members agreed that widespread chronic diseases in the United States require more attention than deficiency diseases, which are rare in the general population. One member was not certain whether the probability approach could be used for chronic diseases. All other members believe it is important to pay continuing attention to the potential for dietary deficiency in the U.S. population.

CONCLUSIONS

The subcommittee has stressed the many important uses of NFCS data. In addition to estimating the prevalence of inadequate intakes, the data permit examination of food use and of dietary patterns. For example, the data are used to establish the patterns of food use associated with nutritional deficiency and with undesirably high levels of nutrient intake (e.g., fat intake). Information about food use, as distinct from nutrient intake, is essential in setting attainable nutritional standards for food assistance programs, for designing meal patterns to meet these programs, and for designing and implementing nutrition education and other nutrition intervention programs intended to ameliorate nutritional problems detected by whatever means in the U.S. population or groups at particular risk. Information about food consumption is essential also in the development of food safety regulations. Thus the NFCS data base is important in supporting many national activities mandated by law. There is no clear replacement, now or in the future, for NFCS data for these types of users.

In recommending design and interpretational enhancements for assessing the prevalence of inadequate intakes, the subcommittee recognizes that this is but one use of the NFCS and not necessarily the most vital use. Therefore, it has repeatedly cautioned that all uses of the data should be considered in making final survey design decisions.

The subcommittee was specifically required by its mandate to evaluate methods to assess observed dietary intake. All except one member of the subcommittee believed that for several nutrients, it should be possible to apply the probability approach, as recommended, at this time.

All the above limitations to the immediate application of the probability approach apply just as much to any other analytical method that is based on a comparison of intakes to requirements (e.g., use of RDA-based cutoffs, nutrient density). Furthermore, to be applied properly, these other methods would also require even more information than the probability approach and this information may be even more difficult to obtain. For this reason, the probability approach has been identified as the preferred method.

After examining the use of fixed cutoff points to analyze dietary adequacy, the subcommittee concluded that attempts to estimate absolute prevalence of inadequate intake using the RDAs or any fixed proportion thereof have no scientific validity and that the results of this type of analysis cannot be meaningfully interpreted. The one exception to this conclusion is analysis for nutrients for which the entire or almost the entire distribution of usual intake is above the RDA. In such cases, it is possible to conclude that inadequate intake is not a major public health problem for that particular nutrient and category of age and sex.

All the recommendations of the subcommittee can be implemented immediately or as a part of a phased approach to implementation. The interpretational approach does not mandate major changes in survey design and therefore should not delay the survey itself. However, the interpretation of the data requires development of the average requirement estimates needed to implement the probability approach. This is beyond the mandate of the subcommittee and could be a task for the National Research Council's Committee on Dietary Allowances. Some preparatory work can be initiated immediately by the USDA. Sensitivity analyses to determine which error sources have a meaningful impact on estimates of prevalence of inadequate intakes, as exemplified within the present report, are recommended for continuation through the next few years. These would serve to resolve disagreements of opinion about the importance of different potential sources of error. More focused sensitivity analyses for nutrients with a potential for having an important impact will guide the longer term research efforts needed for a full application of the approach.

Appropriately analyzed, dietary data can be used as a basis for judging the presumed adequacy of intake. The subcommittee has proposed an appropriate approach to such interpretation. This application is distinct from an assessment of the state of health consequent to inadequate intake. As discussed in a previous report (NRC, 1984), biochemical and clinical observations included in other national surveys are more appropriate for the assessment of nutritional status per se. Nevertheless, dietary data, such as those collected in NFCS, are required in inferring a dietary causation of observed health effects and in considering dietary actions that might ameliorate them.

References

Anderson, G. H., E. T. S. Li, and T. Glanville. 1984. Brain mechanisms and the quantitative and qualitative aspects of food intake. Brain Res. Bull. 12:167-173.

Balogh, M., H. A. Kahn, and J. H. Medalie. 1971. Random repeat 24-hour dietary recalls. Am. J. Clin. Nutr. 24: 304-310.

Beal, V. A., and M. J. Laus, eds. 1982. Proceedings of the Symposium on Dietary Data Collection, Analysis, and Significance. Sponsored by the Department of Food Science and Nutrition, June 15-16, 1981. Research Bulletin No. 675. Massachusetts Agricultural Experiment Station, College of Food and Natural Resources, University of Massachusetts at Amherst.

Beaton, G. H. 1971. The use of nutritional requirements and allowances. Pp. 356-363 in P. L. White and N. Selvey, eds. Proceedings of the Western Hemisphere Nutrition Congress III. Futura Publishing, Mount Kisco, New York.

Beaton, G. H. 1974. Epidemiology of iron deficiency. Pp. 477-528 in A. Jacobs and M. Worwood, eds. Iron in Biochemistry and Medicine. Academic Press, New York.

Beaton, G. H. 1982a. Diet-plasma lipid relationships within a free-living population. Editorial. Arteriosclerosis 2:500-501.

Beaton, G. H. 1982b. What do we think we are estimating? Pp. 36-48 in V. A. Beal and M. J. Laus, eds. Proceedings of the Symposium on Dietary Data Collection, Anal-

ysis, and Significance. Sponsored by the Department
of Food Science and Nutrition, June 15-16, 1981.
Research Bulletin No. 675. Massachusetts Agricultural Experiment Station, College of Food and Natural
Resources, University of Massachusetts at Amherst.

Beaton, G. H. 1983. Energy in human nutrition: Perspec-
tives and problems. Nutr. Rev. 41:325-340.

Beaton, G. H., J. Milner, P. Corey, V. McGuire, M. Cousins,
E. Stewart, M. de Ramos, D. Hewitt, P. V. Grambsch,
N. Kassim, and J. A. Little. 1979. Sources of vari-
ance in 24-hour dietary recall data: Implications for
nutrition study design and interpretation. Am. J.
Clin. Nutr. 32:2546-2559.

Beaton, G. H., J. Milner, V. McGuire, T. E. Feather, and
J. A. Little. 1983. Source of variance in 24-hour
dietary recall data: Implications for nutrition study
design and interpretation. Carbohydrate sources, vitamins, and minerals. Am. J. Clin. Nutr. 37:986-995.

Becker, B. G., B. P. Indik, and A. M. Beeuwkes. 1960.
Dietary Intake Methodologies--A Review. University of
Michigan Research Institute Project 03188. Department
of Public Health Practice, School of Public Health.
University of Michigan, Ann Arbor.

Bickel, P. J., and K. A. Doksum. 1977. Mathematical Statistics: Basic Ideas and Selected Topics. Holden-Day,
San Francisco.

Block, G. 1982. A review of validations of dietary assessment methods. Am. J. Epidemiol. 115:492-505.

Box, G. E. P., and D. R. Cox. 1964. An analysis of transformations. J. R. Stat. Soc. B 26:211-252.

Bray, G. A., B. Zachary, W. T. Dahms, R. L. Atkinson, and
T. H. Oddie. 1978. Eating patterns of massively obese
individuals. J. Am. Diet. Assoc. 72:24-27.

Brownie, C., and J.-P. Habicht. 1984. Selecting a screening cut-off point or diagnostic criterion for comparing
prevalences of disease. Biometrics 40:675-684.

Burk, M. C., and E. M. Pao. 1976. Methodology for Large-Scale Surveys of Household and Individual Diets. Home Economics Research Report No. 40. Agriculture Research Service, U.S. Department of Agriculture, Washington, D.C.

Caliendo, M. A. 1981. Validity of the 24-hour recall to determine dietary status of elderly in an extended care facility. J. Nutr. Elderly 1:57-66.

Campbell, V. A., and M. L. Dodds. 1967. Collecting dietary information from groups of older people. J. Am. Diet. Assoc. 51:29-33.

Comstock, E. M., R. G. St. Pierre, and Y. D. Mackiernan. 1981. Measuring individual plate waste in school lunches. J. Am. Diet. Assoc. 79:290-296.

de St. Jeor, S. T. 1980. Variability in Nutrient Intake: An Appraisal of Food Logs. Ph.D. dissertation. Pennsylvania State University, University Park.

FAO/WHO (Food and Agriculture Organization/World Health Organization). 1967. Requirements of Vitamin A, Thiamine, Riboflavine and Niacin. Report of a Joint FAO/WHO Expert Group. WHO Technical Report Series No. 362. FAO Nutrition Meetings Report Series No. 41. World Health Organization, Geneva.

FAO/WHO (Food and Agriculture Organization/World Health Organization). 1970. Requirements of Ascorbic Acid, Vitamin D, Vitamin B_{12}, Folate, and Iron. Report of a Joint FAO/WHO Expert Group. WHO Technical Report Series No. 452. FAO Nutrition Meetings Report Series No. 47. World Health Organization, Geneva.

FAO/WHO/UNU (Food and Agriculture Organization/World Health Organization/United Nations University). In press. Energy and Protein Requirements. Report of a Joint FAO/WHO/UNU Meeting. World Health Organization, Geneva.

Garn, S. M., F. A. Larkin, and P. E. Cole. 1978. The real problem with 1-day diet records. Letter to the editor. Am. J. Clin. Nutr. 31:1114-1116.

Gersovitz, M., J. P. Madden, and H. Smiciklas-Wright. 1978.
Validity of the 24-hr. dietary recall and seven-day
record for group comparisons. J. Am. Diet. Assoc. 73:
48-55.

Graves, K., and B. Shannon. 1983. Using visual plate waste
measurement to assess school lunch food behavior. J. Am.
Diet. Assoc. 82:163-165.

Greger, J. L., and G. M. Etnyre. 1978. Validity of 24-hour
dietary recalls by adolescent females. Am. J. Publ.
Health 68:70-72.

Guthrie, H. A. 1984. Selection and quantification of
typical food portions by young adults. J. Am. Diet.
Assoc. 84:1440-1444.

Habicht, J.-P. 1980. Some characteristics of indicators of
nutritional status for use in screening and surveillance.
Am. J. Clin. Nutr. 33:531-535.

Habicht, J.-P., L. D. Meyers, and C. Brownie. 1982. Indicators for identifying and counting the improperly nourished. Am. J. Clin. Nutr. 35:1241-1254.

Hackett, A. F., A. J. Rugg-Gunn, and D. R. Appleton. 1983.
Use of a dietary diary and interview to estimate the food
intake of children. Hum. Nutr. Appl. Nutr. 37A:293-300.

Hallfrisch, J., P. Steele, and L. Cohen. 1982. Comparison
of seven-day diet record with measured food intake of
twenty-four subjects. Nutr. Res. 2:263-273.

Hankin, J. H., W. E. Reynolds, and S. Margen. 1967. A
short dietary method for epidemiologic studies. Am. J.
Clin. Nutr. 20:935-945.

Health and Welfare, Canada. 1964. Dietary Standards for
Canada. Canadian Bulletin on Nutrition, Vol. 6, No. 1.
Department of National Health and Welfare, Ottawa.

Health and Welfare, Canada. 1983. Recommended Nutrient
Intakes for Canadians. Compiled by the Committee for
the Revision of the Dietary Standard for Canada. Bureau

of Nutritional Sciences, Food Directorate, Health Protection Branch, Department of National Health and Welfare. Canadian Government Publishing Centre, Ottawa.

Hegsted, D. M. 1972. Problems in the use and interpretation of the Recommended Dietary Allowances. Ecol. Food Nutr. 1:255-265.

Houser, H. B., and H. T. Bebb. 1981. Individual variation in intake of nutrients by day, month, and season and relation to meal patterns: Implications for dietary survey methodology. Pp. 155-179 in Assessing Changing Food Consumption Patterns. A report of the Committee on Food Consumption Patterns, Food and Nutrition Board, Commission on Life Sciences. National Academy Press, Washington, D.C.

Hunt, W. C., A. G. Leonard, P. J. Garry, and J. S. Goodwin. 1983. Components of variance in dietary data for an elderly population. Nutr. Res. 3:433-444.

IUNS (International Union of Nutritional Sciences). 1983a. Recommended Dietary Intakes Around the World, Part I. A report by Committee 1/5 of the International Union of Nutritional Sciences (1982). Nutr. Abstr. Rev. 53: 939-1015.

IUNS (International Union of Nutritional Sciences). 1983b. Recommended Dietary Intakes Around the World, Part II. A report by Committee 1/5 of the International Union of Nutritional Sciences (1982). Nutr. Abstr. Rev. 53: 1075-1119.

Jacobs, D. R., Jr., J. T. Anderson, and H. Blackburn. 1979. Diet and serum cholesterol: Do zero correlations negate the relationship? Am. J. Epidemiol. 110:77-87.

Karvetti, R.-L., and L.-R. Knuts. 1981. Agreement between dietary interviews. J. Am. Diet. Assoc. 79:654-660.

Kato, H., J. Tillotson, M. Z. Nichaman, G. G. Rhoads, and H. B. Hamilton. 1973. Epidemiologic studies of coronary heart disease and stroke in Japanese men living in Japan, Hawaii and California: Serum lipids and diet. Am. J. Epidemiol. 97:372-385.

Keys, A., ed. 1970. Coronary heart disease in seven countries. Circulation 41(4, Suppl. 1):1-199.

Krantzler, N. J., B. J. Mullen, H. G. Schutz, L. E. Grivetti, C. A. Holden, and H. L. Meiselman. 1982. Validity of telephoned diet recalls and records for assessment of individual food intake. Am. J. Clin. Nutr. 36:1234-1242.

Lachance, P. A. 1976. Simple research techniques for school food service. Part II. Measuring plate waste. Sch. Foodserv. J. 30(10):68-72,76.

Lansky, D., and K. D. Brownell. 1982. Estimates of food quantity and calories: Errors in self-report among obese patients. Am. J. Clin. Nutr. 35:727-732.

Linusson, E. E. I., D. Sanjur, and E. C. Erickson. 1975. Validating the 24-hour recall method as a dietary survey tool. Arch. Latinoam. Nutr. 24:277-294.

Liu, K., J. Stamler, A. Dyer, J. McKeever, and P. McKeever. 1978. Statistical methods to assess and minimize the role of intraindividual variability in obscuring the relationship between dietary lipids and serum choles-terol. J. Chronic Dis. 31:399-418.

Lörstad, M. H. 1971. Recommended intake and its relation to nutrient deficiency. FAO Nutr. Newsl. 9:18-31.

Madden, J. P., S. J. Goodman, and H. A. Guthrie. 1976. Validity of the 24-hour recall. J. Am. Diet. Assoc. 68:143-147.

Marr, J. W. 1971. Individual dietary surveys: Purposes and methods. World Rev. Nutr. Diet. 13:105-164.

McGee, D., G. Rhoads, J. Hankin, K. Yano, and J. Tillotson. 1982. Within-person variability of nutrient intake in a group of Hawaiian men of Japanese ancestry. Am. J. Clin. Nutr. 36:657-663.

Meredith, A., A. Matthews, M. Zickefoose, E. Weagley, M. Wayave, and E. G. Brown. 1951. How well do school children recall what they have eaten? J. Am. Diet. Assoc. 27:749-751.

101

Morris, E. R. 1983. An overview of current information on bioavailability of dietary iron to humans. Fed. Proc., Fed. Am. Soc. Exp. Biol. 42:1716-1720.

Morris, J. N., J. W. Marr, J. A. Heady, G. L. Mills, and T. R. E. Pilkington. 1963. Diet and plasma cholesterol in 99 bank men. Br. Med. J. 1:571-576.

Mullen, B. J., N. J. Krantzler, L. E. Grivetti, H. G. Schutz, and H. L. Meiselman. 1984. Validity of a food frequency questionnaire for the determination of individual food intake. Am. J. Clin. Nutr. 39:136-143.

NRC (National Research Council). 1974. Recommended Dietary Allowances, Eighth revised edition. A report of the Committee on Dietary Allowances, Committee on Interpretation of the Recommended Dietary Allowances, Food and Nutrition Board, Assembly of Life Sciences. National Academy of Sciences, Washington, D.C.

NRC (National Research Council). 1980. Recommended Dietary Allowances, Ninth revised edition. A report of the Committee on Dietary Allowances, Food and Nutrition Board, Division of Biological Sciences, Assembly of Life Sciences. National Academy of Sciences, Washington, D.C.

NRC (National Research Council). 1984. National Survey Data on Food Consumption: Uses and Recommendations. A report of the Coordinating Committee on Evaluation of Food Consumption Surveys, Food and Nutrition Board, Commission on Life Sciences. National Academy Press, Washington, D.C.

Pao, E. M., K. H. Fleming, P. M. Guenther, and S. J. Mickle. 1982. Foods Commonly Eaten by Individuals: Amount Per Day and Per Eating Occasion. Home Economics Research Report No. 44. Human Nutrition Information Service, U.S. Department of Agriculture, Washington, D.C.

Pekkarinen, M. 1970. Methodology in the collection of food consumption data. World Rev. Nutr. Diet. 12: 145-171.

Peterkin, B. B., R. L. Kerr, and M. Y. Hama. 1982. Nutritional adequacy of diets of low-income households. J. Nutr. Educ. 14:102-104.

Raker, M. R. 1979. The Validity of a Telephoned Food
    Record. M.S. Thesis. Pennsylvania State University,
    University Park.

Rogan, W. J., and B. Gladen. 1978. Estimating prevalence
    from the results of a screening test. Am. J. Epidemiol.
    107:71-76.

Rush, D., and A. R. Kristal. 1982. Methodologic studies
    during pregnancy: The reliability of the 24-hour dietary
    recall. Am. J. Clin. Nutr. 35:1259-1268.

Schnakenberg, D. D., T. M. Hill, M. J. Kretsch, and B. S.
    Morris. 1981. Diary-interview technique to assess food
    consumption patterns of individual military personnel.
    Pp. 180-197 in Assessing Changing Food Consumption
    Patterns. A report of the Committee on Food Consumption
    Patterns, Food and Nutrition Board, Assembly of Life
    Sciences. National Academy Press, Washington, D.C.

Sempos, C. T., N. E. Johnson, E. L. Smith, and C. Gilligan.
    1985. Effects of intraindividual and interindividual
    variation in repeated dietary records. Am. J. Epidemiol.
    121:120-130.

Sopko, G., D. R. Jacobs, Jr., and H. L. Taylor. 1984.
    Dietary measures of physical activity. Am. J. Epidemiol.
    120:900-911.

Stallones, R. A. 1982. Comments on the assessment of
    nutritional status in epidemiological studies and surveys
    of populations. Am. J. Clin. Nutr. 35:1290-1291.

Stunkard, A. J., and M. Waxman. 1981. Accuracy of self-
    reports of food intake. J. Am. Diet. Assoc. 79:547-551.

Tillotson, J. L., H. Kato, M. Z. Nichaman, D. C. Miller,
    M. L. Gay, K. G. Johnson, and G. G. Rhoads. 1973.
    Epidemiology of coronary heart disease and stroke in
    Japanese men living in Japan, Hawaii, and California:
    Methodology for comparison of diet. Am. J. Clin. Nutr.
    26:177-184.

Todd, K. S., M. Hudes, and D. H. Calloway. 1983. Food
    intake measurement: Problems and appproaches. Am. J.
    Clin. Nutr. 37:139-146.

Trumpler, R. J., and H. F. Weaver. 1953. Statistical
    Astronomy. University of California Press, Berkeley.

USDA (U.S. Department of Agriculture). 1963. Composition
    of Foods: Raw, Processed, Prepared. Agriculture Hand-
    book No. 8. Agricultural Research Service. U.S. Depart-
    ment of Agriculture, Washington, D.C.

USDA (U.S. Department of.Agriculture). 1976-1984.
    Composition of Foods: Raw, Processed, Prepared.
    Agriculture Handbook No. 8, Sect. 1-12. Agricultural
    Research Service, U.S. Department of Agriculture,
    Washington, D.C.

Wolf, W. R. 1981. Assessment of inorganic nutrient intake
    from self-selected diets. Pp. 175-196 in G. R. Beecher,
    ed. Human Nutrition Research. Beltsville Symposia in
    Agricultural Research, 4. Allanheld, Osmun, Totowa, New
    Jersey.

Van Itallie, T. B., and C. E. Woteki. 1985. Health impli-
    cations of overweight and obesity: An American perspec-
    tive. Pp. 15-18 in Health Implications of Obesity. NIH
    Consensus Development Conference, February 11-13, 1985.
    Program and Abstracts.

Young, C. M., F. W. Chalmers, H. N. Church, M. M. Clayton,
    L. O. Gates, G. C. Hagan, B. F. Steele, R. E. Tucker,
    A. W. Wertz, and W. D. Foster. 1952. Subject's ability
    to estimate food portions. Pp. 17-19 in Cooperative
    Nutritional Status Studies in the Northeast Region. III.
    Dietary Methodology Studies. Bulletin No. 469. North-
    east Regional Publication No. 10. University of Massa-
    chusetts Agricultural Experiment Station, Amherst.

Statement Concerning Application of the Recommended Method[1]

D. M. Hegsted

The subcommittee is in agreement that under ideal conditions the probability approach which is recommended appears to offer the best available approach to estimating the proportion of the population at risk of nutritional deficiency from dietary survey data. As the report notes, dietary surveys are used as a basis for determining the magnitude of inadequate nutrition, serve as a basis for food assistance programs, etc., and a general instrument for formulation of nutrition policy. I believe that the recommendation that the probability approach be adopted is premature. The method has not been adequately tested. It appears likely that this approach will grossly overestimate the extent of inadequate nutrition in the country and, thus, lead to inappropriate policy decisions.

The two major requirements for the application of the probability approach are a) that there be available reasonably accurate estimates of the mean requirement for each nutrient and an estimate of the range of requirements within the population group, and b) that the survey methodology yield satisfactory estimates of the usual nutrient intakes of the group.

---

[1]Dissenting statements prepared by individual members of a committee are not subject to the normal National Research Council review processes, nor are they subject to committee or staff editing or review. They appear exactly as the dissenting committee members prepare them. The Research Council neither endorses nor takes responsibility for the content of the statements.

NUTRIENT REQUIREMENT INFORMATION

Currently available estimates of the mean requirement for any nutrient are confined to few age-sex groups,
usually young adult men or women. Presumably the dietary
survey data will be analyzed according to the format of
the Recommended Dietary Allowances which provide values for
17 or more age-sex groups. If so, "requirement curves" for
each nutrient for each of these age-sex groups must be
inferred from the limited data available. Just how this
can be done to yield reliable values is unclear and one
must assume that such derived values will be less accurate
than values based upon actual data.

There are even less data on the range of requirements within any age-sex group. The report places considerable reliance on the assumption that protein requirements determined by nitrogen balance have a standard deviation of about 15% of the mean value. It must be emphasized that this value is the total variance of requirements determined by this technique which includes the
variation due to error as well as biologic variation. It
is the latter which is of importance. Since the estimated
mean requirement for nitrogen balance may vary by as much
as 50% depending upon the experimental protocol, particularly the prior diet of the individual subjects, it is
apparent that the error term must be large and one must
assume that the true biologic variation is relatively
small. In all estimates of the variability in nutrient
requirements derived from compilation of values in the
literature the error term must be similarly large since
the experimental protocol, background of the subjects,
etc., differ.

The other example of differences in requirements is
based upon blood losses in women of the childbearing age
which can be translated into differences in iron requirements. The utility of this example, however, is compro-
mised by many factors which influence iron absorption,
such as the adaptive response of the individual, the form
of iron in the diet, and the amounts of various factors
which promote or inhibit iron absorption. Indeed, it
appears that such factors are more important in determining the availability of iron than the amount of iron
actually consumed. One may make general assumptions about
average levels of iron and of these factors in the diet in
establishing recommended levels of iron intake, but these

have little applicability for the individual. We have no methodology for including these factors in the probability approach, and estimates of the proportion of the population at risk of iron deficiency inevitably suffer. The recent analysis of the extent of iron deficiency in the American population for the NHANES data indicates that the probability approach overestimates the extent of the problem.

Currently available information on the nutritional status of Americans and recent developments in nutrition inevitably shift the interest in dietary surveys and how they should be interpreted. Nutritional deficiency disease is clearly not a major public health problem. The major chronic diseases are the major public health problem, and these are nutrition related. Interest in dietary surveys in the future should focus on these problems rather than nutritional deficiency. Thus, to varying degrees, the report focuses attention on the wrong problem and fails to indicate how the survey data should be examined relative to these more important issues.

Nutritional standards related to excessive consumption of fat, cholesterol, sugar, or salt can probably not be derived by attempting to develop curves related to requirements or toxicity. Rather, these are developed by attempting to accommodate desirability, feasibility, acceptability, etc. Whether approaches similar to those outlined for the probability approach can be adapted to these issues is unclear at this time.

Recent evidence implicates vitamin A, carotene, and vitamin C in the etiology of cancer. If intake of these materials is relevant to cancer, it will have a profound effect upon the interpretation of dietary surveys since even modest effects upon cancer prevalence are immeasurably more important than the defined nutritional deficiencies. Yet the likelihood that one can develop reliable estimates of requirements to prevent cancer seems relatively remote at this time, and the probability approach can probably not be applied.

The subcommittee notes that for a considerable number of nutrients the information on requirements and/or range of requirements is virtually nonexistent, the probability approach cannot be applied, and estimates of the proportion of the population at risk cannot be made. No doubt this

is true, but it seems rather unlikely that these nutrients
can be simply ignored in evaluating dietary survey data.

Finally, the subcommittee recommends that research to
improve knowledge of nutrient requirements be expanded in
order to make the application of the probability approach
more feasible. No doubt this is desirable, but given the
fact that nutritional deficiency does not appear to be a
major public health issue, it is quite unlikely that such
research can be a national research priority except for a
few nutrients. Thus it seems unlikely that the necessary
data required for more accurate application of the probability approach will be available any time in the near
future.

ESTIMATES OF NUTRIENT INTAKE

The report recognizes that the reporting of food intake
is subject to gross errors but, in my opinion, fails to
adequately consider the impact of such errors on the reliability of the estimated extent of malnutrition. The
application of the probability approach rests upon the
assumption that the errors in reported food intake and
calculated nutrient intake are randomly distributed, i.e.,
that it is equally likely that under- and overreporting
occur with equal frequency and extent. No doubt the
reliability of the data collected in any survey will
depend upon the methodology used, but most of the data
available do not support the supposition and, even if it
is true that mean intakes are correctly reported (over-
and underreporting are equal), the method will still
apparently overestimate the extent of undernutrition.

Chapter 6 refers to many of the reports which have
attempted to validate the reliability of dietary recall or
food records. While the conclusions vary, a large number
of investigators find that such methods often yield grossly
low estimates of energy consumption, in some cases to the
surprising extent of 30 to 40 percent underestimate.
It should be noted that most such estimates refer to energy
intake only. It can be assumed that total energy intake
will be similar whether the subjects are free-living or
under controlled conditions if weight is maintained and
physical activity is similar. It is much more difficult,
or perhaps impossible, to obtain reliable estimates of
intake of other nutrients in free-living subjects. It is

reasonable to assume that most subjects will be more likely
to forget to recall or record food eaten than they will
list foods not eaten. Furthermore, most of the literature
reports have obviously been obtained with relatively well-
motivated subjects. This cannot be assumed in large scale
surveys where motivation may be minimal, and instructions
to the subjects will generally be less extensive than in
well-designed studies.

However, even if the mean intake of a group is correctly recorded, it still seems likely that the probability approach will yield excessive estimates of the
extent of malnutrition. It is certain that a substantial
part of the survey population will underestimate their
individual average intake either because of error or
because the two or three days during which intake is
measured were atypically low. When nutrient intakes vary
greatly from one day to the next as they do in the U.S.,
often 100%, it is inevitable that a substantial number of
atypical intakes will be recorded. The probability
approach (or any other approach that has been suggested)
is concerned only with the number of low intakes, the
"tail end" of the distribution of intakes. These remain
to be counted as in risk of deficiency even though overestimates might yield a correct mean value for the group.

The calculation of "usual intakes" by subtracting the
intraindividual variance from the total variance no doubt
diminishes the extent of erroneously recorded low intakes,
but when data are available for only two or three days, it
is not eliminated. The consumption, for example, of a
potent source of carotenoids once a week might provide an
adequate intake of vitamin A.

Another criticism of the probability approach is that
it provides no estimate of the severity of deficiency.
Subjects whose consumption is only modestly below standard
are grouped with those well below standard. The report
recommends that multiple standards be applied in order to
provide an estimate of severity but, at this time, only
the RDAs are available as standards. We can anticipate
obvious problems if agencies establish their own "requirement curves" to meet their own needs or expectations.

CONCLUSION

It appears to me that the probability approach rests upon a weak foundation both with respect to the data on nutrient requirements and, especially, the survey methodology. Most of the errors, biases, and variability in the data collected are likely to result in substantial overestimates of the extent of undernutrition. The calculated examples in the body of the report do not appear to be reassuring since, except for protein, they indicate large numbers at risk of apparently all other nutrients examined. This seems inconsistent with the reasonably well-based conclusion that nutritional deficiencies are not a public health problem of any magnitude in this country.

The probability approach gives the impression that the estimates of undernutrition are rather precise since the utility of the extensive statistical calculations is not apparent otherwise. The identification of such "problems" will presumably call for public health solutions. Unless the "problems" are real, which I doubt, this will result in large expenditures of money and effort with little or no benefit. Indeed, no solution appears to be in sight nor are there other data indicating that the problems exist.

Dietary surveys are useful in indicating food patterns and provide data for rough comparisons of differences between groups, time trends in food consumption, etc. Until some data are available which indicate that the estimates of undernutrition obtained by application of the probability approach are available, however, I do not believe we should recommend its application. The most appropriate recommendations of the subcommittee should be that the probability approach deserves further study but, at this time, the extent of under- or malnutrition can not be determined from dietary survey data.

Adjustment of Intake Distributions Used in This Report

All original analyses in this report have been based on data from the 1977-1978 Nationwide Food Consumption Survey (NFCS), which were provided by the U.S. Department of Agriculture (USDA) for this purpose. Data were available for approximately 2,400 women and 1,750 men between the ages of 23 and 34 years.

As described in Chapter 4, food intakes estimated on each of 3 consecutive days were not collected by the same technique each day. The first method of observation consisted of an interview and recall of foods eaten on the day prior to the interview. The respondent was then instructed to keep a record of food intake for the remainder of the day of the interview and the following day. Subsequent statistical analyses have suggested that either the method or the sequence of observation days has an effect on reported intake; however, this effect has not been considered in the analysis presented herein. The resulting variance has been pooled with intraindividual variance. Because the data refer to adjacent days rather than to independent estimates of intake, there is a potential for loss of statistical power as a result of the design of data collection, because of possible correlation of food intake between days for a given person.

Note: The data analyzed in this report are for nutrients ingested in foods. Information about dietary supplements was not included in the 1977-1978 NFCS. As a result, all analyses presented in the report underestimate intake and overestimate the prevalence of inadequate intake. The magnitude of this bias is not known.

The USDA provided data in the form of fixed frequency interval distributions. The data for individual
subjects were ranked and the mean intake computed for
each interval. Altogether there were 200 intervals,
each consisting of 0.5% of the subject days. The data
were presented in three ways: (1) data for 1 day without grouping data for each person (i.e., as if all data
were independent), (2) mean values for 3 days of intake
data for each person, and (3) mean values of the loga-
rithm of intakes for each of 3 days for each person.
These were the basic working data sets for the analyses
presented in this report.

The USDA also conducted and reported to the subcommittee its analysis of variance (ANOVA) results for the
NFCS data. For this analysis, the 1-day data were logarithmically transformed, and the subcommittee performed
an ANOVA by standard techniques, assigning variance to
model (subjects), to day (sequence), and to residual.
Subsequently, variance was assigned to only two
components--model and residual. A typical ANOVA is
displayed in Table A-1, together with an illustration of
the derivation of interindividual and intraindividual
variance estimates. From the data transformation shown
in the table, the variance attributable to subjects is
computed as:

V(subject) = (0.40930366 - 0.16502502)/3 = 0.081427866,
and the standard deviations (SDs) attributable to subjects
(interindividual) and to day-to-day variation within subjects

TABLE A-1. ANOVA: Protein Intake by Adult Men, Shown by
Logarithmically Transformed Data

Source	Degrees of Freedom	Sum of Squares	Mean Square
Model[a]	1,751	716.69947157	0.40930866
Error[b]	3,498	577.25751426	0.16502502
Total[c]	5,249	1,293.95698583	

[a] 3 V(subject) + V(error).
[b] V(error).
[c] Corrected.

(intraindividual) are computed as the square roots of
V(subject) and V(error). Thus, SD(inter) = 0.2853556 and
SD(intra) = 0.4062326. The adjusted SD of 3-day data may be
estimated as the square root of the sum of variances
[V(subject) + V(error)]/3 to yield a 3-day SD of 0.369372.

The results of ANOVAs carried out for the NFCS data sets
are presented in Table A-2. For comparison, the observed
SDs in the original logarithmically transformed data sets
are presented as well as the 3-day SD derived as described
above.

In estimating the distribution of usual intakes, the
objective was to remove the effects of the day-to-day
variation in intake, the error term in the ANOVA. This
component of variation includes both real day-to-day
variation in intake and any random error in methodology
(e.g., day-to-day variation in under- and overreporting of
actual intake attributable to method). Of course, it does
not adjust for any systematic bias in the data sets (consistent under- or overreporting for individual subjects).

TABLE A-2. Estimates of Interindividual and Intraindividual Variation in Logarithmically
Transformed Data[a]

| Nutrient | Estimates of Variation | | |
	Number of Subjects	SD(inter-individual)	SD(intra-individual)
Males:			
Protein	1,752	0.2853	0.4062
Iron	1,752	0.2909	0.3825
Vitamin A	1,752	0.5119	0.8547
Vitamin B	1,752	0.6493	0.8441
Thiamin/day	1,752	0.3497	0.4415
Thiamin/kcal	1,752	0.1898	0.3421
Females:			
Protein	2,394	0.3370	0.4468
Iron	2,394	0.3518	0.3987
Vitamin A	2,394	0.6092	0.8834
Vitamin C	2,394	0.7090	0.8843

[a]Derived from the subcommittee's analysis of the 1977-
1978 NFCS.

If all data sets fit perfectly to the normal distribution, it would be possible to use the mean and interindividual SD to completely describe the new distribution. However, examination of the distributions revealed a number of departures from normality. An approach that was adopted might preserve some of the uniqueness of the original distribution while removing the effect of intraindividual variation. This approach is described by the following algorithm, which was applied to each interval of intake in the original transformed data set:

Adjusted intake = (observed intake - mean intake)
$$\text{x } \frac{\text{SD(interindividual)}}{\text{SD(observed)}} + \text{mean intake.}$$

This adjustment created a new distribution with 200 intervals, still in logarithmically transformed form. By computing the exponential of the values, the distribution was converted back to the original units and could then be used in subsequent computations as an estimate of the distribution of usual intakes.

Descriptive information on some of the distributions used in this report is presented in Table A-3. The 1-day intake distribution consists of all single-day measurements analyzed as if they were independent observations. The 3-day intake distribution represents the means, calculated at the level of individuals, for three replicates of intake. The logarithmically transformed 3-day distribution represents the mean log of each day calculated at the level of the individual. The transformed distribution, in original units, is as described above. The most critical measure in the data presented is the degree to which the transformed data fit the normal assumption. It would have been preferable to develop a transformation algorithm appropriate to the individual data set before conducting the ANOVA (Box and Cox, 1964). However, this exercise was not conducted for the present report.

REFERENCES

Box, G. E. P., and D. R. Cox. 1964. An analysis of transformations. J. R. Stat. Soc. B26:211-252.

Cochran, W. G., and G. W. Snedecor. 1980. Statistical Methods, Seventh edition. Iowa State University Press, Ames.

TABLE A-3. Characteristics of the Distributions of Nutrient Intake in This Report

Nutrient and Data Set	Mean	Median	Observed SD	Skew[a]	Kurtosis[b]
MALES:					
Protein (g/day)					
1-day data	97.8	91.4	45.0	1.185	3.021
3-day data	97.8	93.9	33.9	1.038	2.639
Transformed data	4.4744	4.503	0.3695	-0.571	1.273
Adjusted data	91.2	89.6	25.0	0.578	1.308
Iron (mg/day)					
1-day data	15.9	14.7	7.4	1.369	3.820
3-day data	15.9	15.1	5.7	1.302	3.880
Transformed data	2.6570	2.676	0.3655	-0.335	0.849
Adjusted data	14.9	14.5	4.3	0.849	2.046
Vitamin A (IU/day)					
1-day data	5,570	3,375	9,125	7.939	82.743
3-day data	5,600	4,155	5,800	4.645	30.160
Transformed data	8.1160	8.150	0.7194	-0.525	1.152
Adjusted data	3,780	3.420	1.890	1.411	3.594
Vitamin C (mg/day)					
1-day data	85.2	57.0	84.6	2.279	7.869
3-day data	85.3	66.7	67.5	2.072	6.630
Transformed data	3.9391	3.980	0.8770	-0.372	0.118
Adjusted data	62.4	52.8	39.4	1.476	3.297
Thiamin (mg/day)					
1-day data	1.53	1.36	0.87	1.596	4.012
3-day data	1.54	1.44	0.67	1.494	4.422
Transformed data	0.2797	0.310	0.4334	-0.234	0.516
Adjusted data	1.40	1.35	0.49	1.135	2.903
Thiamin (mg/1,000 kcal)					
1-day data	0.64	0.59	0.27	1.570	3.862
3-day data	0.64	0.62	0.18	1.095	2.837
Transformed data	-0.5175	-0.521	0.2738	-0.179	1.232
Adjusted data	0.61	0.60	0.12	0.697	1.914
FEMALES:					
Protein (g/day)					
1-day data	65.5	61.6	31.1	0.918	1.605
3-day data	65.6	63.0	24.1	0.787	1.264
Transformed data	4.0527	4.097	0.4377	-1.277	4.469
Adjusted data	61.3	59.5	18.3	0.346	0.682
Iron (mg/day)					
1-day data	10.8	10.0	5.3	1.367	3.800
3-day data	10.8	10.2	4.2	1.318	3.962
Transformed data	2.2567	2.290	0.4195	-0.848	2.796
Adjusted data	10.2	9.8	3.3	0.812	2.088
Vitamin A (IU/day)					
1-day data	4,620	2,740	7,360	6.605	58.298
3-day data	4,690	3,340	5,065	3.911	20.675
Transformed data	7.8647	7.916	0.8488	-0.853	2.472
Adjusted data	3,160	2,700	1,800	1.519	3.891
Vitamin C (mg/day)					
1-day data	73.1	48.0	72.9	1.933	5.440
3-day data	72.6	57.3	56.8	1.509	2.872
Transformed data	3.7219	3.785	0.9789	-0.528	0.438
Adjusted data	52.8	43.1	34.8	1.316	2.312

[a]Algorithms for skew calculations from Cochran and Snedecor, 1980, pp. 78-79.
[b]From Cochran and Snedecor, 1980, pp. 79-81.

APPENDIX *B*

Derivation of Criteria for Interpreting Iron Intake in Women

As discussed in Chapter 5, when nutrient requirements are symmetrically distributed around the mean, the
probability assessment approach is relatively insensitive to the shape of the requirement distribution. This
is not true when the distribution is markedly asymmetrical, as for iron requirements of menstruating women.
For this reason, it is important to estimate the characteristics of the distribution of iron requirements for
this group.

In agreement with the FAO/WHO Expert Group (FAO/WHO,
1970), the iron losses are divided into two components:
basal losses via the skin, urine, and feces (excreted
iron rather than unabsorbed iron) and the losses in the
menses. The need for absorbed iron to balance these
losses is then estimated using the upper limit of
absorption of dietary iron that can be expected in
persons ingesting a mixed diet, who are in need of iron,
but maintaining body iron stores. The development of
these components of the final estimate is described
below.

An isotopic technique has been used to measure basal
iron losses for adult men under various conditions
(Green et al., 1968). For the purpose of this appendix,
the data obtained with this technique have been extrapo-
lated to women on the basis of relative metabolic size,
as reflected by basal metabolic rate (BMR). The mean
basal iron loss derived in this manner is approximately
0.67 mg/day. There are few data on the variability of
these losses, other than those in the original studies
of men. A coefficient of variation (CV) of approximately 15% used for this exercise results in a range

115

from about 0.47 to 0.87 mg/day. For simplicity, a basal loss of 0.87 mg/day was accepted for all women--a small overestimation of actual need.

Iron content of the menses is the major factor affecting the distribution of iron needs among menstruating women. Several studies have established that there is considerable variation among women but a similarity from cycle to cycle for individual women. Thus, losses for a population of women should be fairly similar to the distribution of iron requirements used in the probability approach. Suitable data on iron losses have been provided in the reports of two large population studies (Cole et al., 1971; Hallberg et al., 1966), which are supported by the findings from a number of smaller studies (see Beaton, 1974). A simple examination of the distribution of observed iron losses would lead to an underestimate of both loss and requirements of women replete with iron because women with high blood losses tend to have low hemoglobin levels (i.e., a tendency toward anemia). To circumvent this, the distribution of blood losses was converted to iron losses by using a standard hemoglobin concentration rather than the hemoglobin level of the study subject. The resultant distributions for the two studies were then merged and found to be in good agreement. A log-normal distribution model that fit the data reasonably well (Beaton, 1974) was used for modeling. Expressed in terms of natural logarithms, the menstrual iron loss distribution may be described as having a mean of -0.81 and a standard deviation of 0.84.

Iron absorption is a regulated process, and within the limits of bioavailability of dietary iron, the body will absorb sufficient iron to meet one's needs and will reject (i.e., absorb with lower efficiency) iron above these needs. Since the objective is to estimate the lowest intake of dietary iron that will maintain iron balance in relation to known losses, there is a need to estimate the upper limit of iron absorption. As iron depletion increases, the efficiency of iron absorption also increases.

After reviewing various kinds of information, the FAO/WHO (1970) committee suggested that the upper limit of absorption was approximately 20% among subjects consuming diets relatively rich in meat and other animal proteins. Since the nature of different diets affects iron bioavailability (Monsen et al., 1978), the upper limit suggested by the FAO/WHO committee was much lower for subjects consuming predominantly cereal diets. The 20% upper limit absorption figure is appreciably higher than the commonly quoted average iron absorption of adult men. Nonetheless, it has been used in the models presented in this report. To examine the effect of defining the requirement in terms of some iron-depleted state (e.g., mild anemia), one need only alter the estimate of the upper limit of iron absorption by increasing it.

To apply this model in the assessment of intake, the following algorithms were adopted:

Available iron = OI x UL, where OI = observed intake (mean intake for the frequency interval) and UL = upper limit of absorption, i.e., 20% for the iron replete state.

Iron available to meet menstrual loss = (OI x UL) - 0.87, where 0.87 mg/day is the assumed basal loss of iron (see comments above), and the position in the normal distribution (Z score) is calculated as:

$$Z = \frac{Ln\ [(OI\ x\ UL) - 0.87] - (-0.81),}{0.84}$$

where -0.81 is the mean of the distribution of logarithms of menstrual iron losses, 0.84 is the standard deviation of that distribution, and the probability that the observed intake would be inadequate to meet iron losses is computed by an algorithm describing the cumulative area under the normal distribution curve to the right of Z. This phase of the calculation is identical with that used for nonlogarithmic distribution models.

Beaton (1974) attempted to validate this model by comparing predicted prevalences of inadequate intake with predicted response to iron administration. He based the latter on the probability of response associated with observed hematocrit, using data from a population study by Garby et al. (1969a,b). There was reasonable agreement when hematologic data from Nutrition Canada and from the Ten-State Nutrition Survey were examined by a probability approach and then compared with assessments based on dietary data from 1-week studies. The model described above has been used to estimate dietary iron requirements in the recent revision of Recommended Nutrient Intakes for Canadians, which contains further discussion on this topic (Health and Welfare, Canada, 1983). With this model, the current Canadian recommended

intake of iron (14 mg/day) would be adequate to meet the
needs of all but approximately 5% of menstruating women,
whereas the U.S. recommended intake (18 mg/day) would meet
the predicted needs of all but about 2% to 3% of women.

REFERENCES

Beaton, G. H. 1974. Epidemiology of iron deficiency.
Pp. 477-528 in A. Jacobs and M. Worwood, eds. Iron in
Biochemistry and Medicine. Academic Press, New York.

Cole, S. K., W. Z. Billewicz, and A. M. Thomson. 1971.
Sources of variation in menstrual blood loss. J. Obstet.
Gynaecol. Br. Commonw. 78:933-939.

FAO/WHO (Food and Agriculture Organization/World Health
Organization). 1970. Requirements of Ascorbic Acid,
Vitamin D, Vitamin B_{12}, Folate, and Iron. Report of a
Joint FAO/WHO Expert Group. WHO Technical Report Series
No. 452. FAO Nutrition Meetings Report Series No. 47.
World Health Organization, Geneva.

Garby, L., L. Irnell, and I. Werner. 1969a. Iron deficiency in women of fertile age in a Swedish community.
II. Efficiency of several laboratory tests to predict
the response to iron supplementation. Acta Med. Scand.
185:107-111.

Garby, L., L. Irnell, and I. Werner. 1969b. Iron deficiency in women of fertile age in a Swedish community.
III. Estimation of prevalence based on response to iron
supplementation. Acta Med. Scand. 185:113-117.

Green, R., R. Charlton, H. Seftel, T. Bothwell, F. Mayet,
B. Adams, C. Finch, and M. Layrisse. 1968. Body iron
excretion in man: A collaborative study. Am. J. Med.
45:336-353.

Hallberg, L., A.-M. Högdahl, L. Nilsson, and G. Rybo. 1966.
Menstrual blood loss--a population study: Variation at
different ages and attempts to define normality. Acta
Obstet. Gynaecol. Scand. 45:320-351.

Health and Welfare, Canada. 1983. Recommended Nutrient
Intakes for Canadians. Compiled by the Committee for
the Revision of the Dietary Standard for Canada. Bureau
of Nutritional Sciences, Food Directorate, Health Protection Branch, Department of National Health and
Welfare. Canadian Government Publishing Centre, Ottawa.

Monsen, E. R., L. Hallberg, M. Layrisse, D. M. Hegsted,
J. D. Cook, W. Mertz, and C. A. Finch. 1978. Estimation of available dietary iron. Am. J. Clin. Nutr.
31:134-141.

Method of Estimating Confidence Intervals

Two specific elements are necessary for the probability approach: a distribution of required intake for a population and a distribution of actual intake. It is also assumed that required intake and actual intake are independent.

DESCRIPTION OF METHOD

The random variable X describes required intake with a distribution function:

$$G(x) = P(X \leq x).$$

Let the random variable Y describe the actual intake with a distribution function:

$$F(x) = P(Y \leq x).$$

The proportion of persons with inadequate intake can be expressed as the proportion of people whose actual intake is below the required intake:

$$P(Y \leq X).$$

This can be written as $\int_{-\infty}^{\infty} P[X \geq y | Y = y] dF(y)$, where $P(A|B)$ corresponds to the conditional probability of event A, given event B.

Under the assumption that X and Y are independent,

$$P[X \geq y | Y = y] = P[X \geq y] = 1 - G(y),$$

and hence

$$P[Y \leq X] = \int [1 - G(y)] dF(y) = 1 - \int G(y) dF(y).$$

The estimate for the distribution of actual intakes, $F(x)$ (described below), is based on survey data of individual daily intakes. Because daily intakes for any given person vary from day to day, this implies that the same person might on some days be above and on other days be below his or her required intake simply because of day-to-day variability. Presumably then, usual intake, an idealized average intake of persons over a long period, is of interest.

Therefore, $F(x)$ should represent the distribution of these idealized averages for a population. To compute $F(x)$ in this manner, one must separate the intraindividual variability from the idealized interindividual variability.

ESTIMATING THE DISTRIBUTION OF ACTUAL INTAKES $F(x)$

The Parametric Method

The data are first transformed to approximate normality. For this purpose, the log transformation seems to work well for most nutrients, but not for all.

A random components model is then fitted to the transformed data. The term y_{ij} denotes the observation of intake for the jth replication of the ith individual, where $i = 1, \ldots, I$, and $j = 1, \ldots, J$. The transformation function is denoted by $g(.)$, and the transformed data are denoted by $z_{ij} = g(y_{ij})$. The random components model is given by

$$z_{ij} = \mu + \alpha_i + e_{ij},$$

where α_i is assumed to be identically and independently distributed (iid) $N(0, \sigma_A^2)$ and the e_{ij} are assumed to be independent $[N(0, \sigma_e^2)]$. The variance σ_e^2 refers to the intraindividual variability, and σ_A^2 refers to the interindividual variability.

If the intraindividual variability were eliminated, then the distribution of $Z = g(Y)$ would be distributed as a normal distribution with mean μ and variance σ_A^2, both of which can be estimated efficiently by the sample mean and the results of a 1-way ANOVA as described in Chapter 4.

In this approach, the distribution of idealized actual intakes is given by $F(x) = P(Y \leq x)$. Hence,

$$P[g(Y) \leq g(x)] = \int_{-\infty}^{g(x)} (2\pi\sigma_A^2)^{-1/2} \exp\{-1/2[g(y) - \mu]^2/\sigma_A^2\}dy.$$

Therefore,

$$dF(x) = (2\pi\sigma_A^2)^{-1/2} \exp\{-1/2[g(x) - \mu]^2/\sigma_A^2\}g'(x)dx,$$

where $g'(x) = dg(x)/dx$.

The proportion of persons with inadequate intakes is given by $1 - K(\mu,\sigma_A^2) = \int G(x)(2\pi\sigma_A^2)^{-1/2}\exp-1/2\{[g(x) - \mu]^2\sigma_A^2\}g'(x)dx$. Hence, we can estimate $K(\mu,\sigma_A^2)$ by $K(\hat{\mu},\hat{\sigma}_A^2)$, where

$$\hat{\mu} = z.. = \sum_{i=1}^{I} \sum_{j=1}^{J} z_{ij}/IJ, \text{ and } \hat{\sigma}_A^2 = J^{-1}(MS_A - MS_e),$$

where $MS_A = J\sum_i(z_i. - z..)^2/(I - 1)$ and $MS_e = \sum_i \sum_j (z_{ij} - z_i.)^2/I(J - 1)$.

In a balanced 1-way random components model, the estimates for the second moments of $\hat{\mu}$ and $\hat{\sigma}_A^2$ are given by:

$$\hat{Var}(\hat{\mu}) = (MS_A)/IJ,$$
$$\hat{Var}(\hat{\sigma}_A^2) = 2J^{-2}\{(I - 1)^{-1} MS_A^2 + [I(J - 1)]^{-1} MS_e^2\}, \text{ and}$$
$$Cov(\hat{\mu},\hat{\sigma}_A^2) = 0.$$

Because $K(\mu,\sigma_A^2)$ is a smooth function of μ and σ_A^2, and for large samples the estimates $\hat{\mu}$ and $\hat{\sigma}_A^2$ are asymptotically normal, the 95% confidence interval can be approximated using the delta method (Bickel and Doksum, 1977). That is, the 95% confidence interval is approximately given by:

$$K(\hat{\mu},\sigma_A^2) \pm 2S_K,$$

where $S_K^2 = [\dfrac{\partial K(\hat{\mu},\hat{\sigma}_A^2)}{\partial \mu}]^2 \hat{Var}(\hat{\mu}) + [\dfrac{\partial K(\hat{\mu},\hat{\sigma}_A^2)}{\partial \sigma_A^2}]^2 (\hat{Var})(\hat{\sigma}_A^2).$

The partial derivatives would be calculated most easily using numerical methods. That is,

$$\frac{\partial K}{\partial \mu} = \frac{K(\hat{\mu} + h,\hat{\sigma}_A^2) - K(\hat{\mu} - h,\hat{\sigma}_A^2)}{2h},$$

given that h is sufficiently small. Similarly,

$$\frac{\partial K}{\partial \sigma_A^2} = \frac{K(\hat{\mu},\hat{\sigma}_A^2 + h) - K(\hat{\mu},\hat{\sigma}_A^2 - h)}{2h}.$$

The parametric approach can be used as long as the distribution of the transformed data is approximately normal. If not, a larger class of transformations such as the Box-Cox (power) transformation, should be considered (Box and Cox, 1964).

The data can be plotted on normal probability graph paper, and formal goodness-of-fit tests can be performed to determine if the transformed data are sufficiently close to normality to make the method valid (Hoaglin and Mosteller, 1982).

The Nonparametric Approach

To implement the probability approach, we must have an estimate of the distribution of actual intake in a specified population, F*(x). Since nutritional intake of individuals varies from day to day, it is assumed that a person's intake corresponds to an idealized average intake over a long period. Let Y_{ij} denote the amount of nutrient ingested by individual i on day j. We assume that some transformation of Y_{ij}, say Z_{ij}, follows a random components model. That is, $Z_{ij} = d_i + e_{ij}$ and $Z_{ij} = g(Y_{ij})$, where the d_i are iid with distribution function F*, and Z_{ij} are assumed to be iid with distribution function G and are independent of the d_i. The distribution function G is assumed to have a mean equal to zero and a variance of σ_e^2 (intraindividual variability), whereas the distribution F* (distribution of idealized average of transformed intakes) has a mean of μ and a variance of σ_A^2 (interindividual variation).

The sample averages $Z_i. = \sum_{j=1}^{J} Z_{ij}/J = d_i + e_i$ has distribution function H, a mean of μ, and a variance of $\sigma_A^2 + \sigma_e^2/J = \sigma^2_{obs}$, where σ^2_{obs} is the estimated SD for the observed sample averages. In the above parametric approach, the underlying distributions $\hat{F}*$ and G were assumed to follow a normal density. The subcommittee believes that without making any specific parametric assumptions about the underlying distribution of F*, a reasonable estimate of F* can be obtained by assuming that the shape of the distribution function of F* should be similar to that of H. This motivated the heuristic estimate of F*, which takes the shape of the empirical cdf,

$$\hat{H}(x) = \sum_{i=1}^{n} I(Z_i. \leq x)/n,$$

where $I = (Z_i. \leq x) = \{ \begin{matrix} 1 \\ 0 \end{matrix}$ if $\begin{matrix} Z_i. \leq x \\ Z_i. > x \end{matrix} \}$

and shrinks it toward the mean. The scaled estimate $\hat{F}*_{(x)} = \hat{H}[\hat{\mu} + (x - \hat{\mu})\hat{\sigma}_{obs}/\hat{\sigma}_A]$ has the following properties:

• The mean is equal to $\hat{\mu}$.

• The variance is equal to $\hat{\sigma}_A^2$ (estimate of interindividual variability).

• The shape of $\hat{F}*$ resembles that of $\hat{H}$.

This estimate was chosen on a heuristic basis and should be a reasonable approximation to F*. Strictly speaking, it is really not a nonparametric estimate in that $\hat{F}*$ will be a consistent estimate of F* for only restricted cases (i.e., if F* were normal); however, we believe it will serve as a reasonable approximation for skewed distributions as well.

Therefore, an estimate for $F(x) - P[Y \leq x]$ can be taken as $= P[g(Y) \leq g(x)] = \hat{H} g\{\mu + (x - \mu) \sigma_{obs}/\sigma_A\}$ and the estimate for the proportion of individuals with inadequate intake would be:

$$\int G(x) d\hat{H}[g\{\hat{\mu} + (x - \hat{\mu}) \frac{\hat{\sigma}_{obs}}{\hat{\sigma}_A}\}].$$

The distributional properties for the nonparametric method are more complicated than the parametric approach because no implicit assumption of normality can be made. For this reason, a bootstrap distribution is used to calculate the confidence interval. This is performed as follows:

1. I individuals are sampled at random with replacement from the I group in the original data set to create a simulated data set:

$$(z_{R1}, j, j = 1, \ldots, J), (z_{R2}, j, j = 1, \ldots, J), \ldots,$$
$$(z_{RI}, j, j = 1, \ldots, J),$$

where $R_1, \ldots, R_I$ are random indices from 1 to I chosen with equal probability.

2. With this simulated data set, an empirical cdf $\hat{H}^B(x)$ is computed and an ANOVA is performed on the simulated data to compute $\hat{\mu}^B$, $\hat{\sigma}^B_{obs}$, and $\hat{\sigma}^B_A$.

3. Then an estimate for the proportion with inadequate intake is computed in the following manner:

$$\int G(x) d\hat{H}^B[g\{\hat{\mu}^B + (x - \hat{\mu}^B) \frac{\hat{\sigma}^B_{obs}}{\hat{\sigma}^B_A}\}].$$

4. Steps 1 through 3 are repeated with random sets of simulated data to generate a distribution of the prevalence of inadequate intake. The confidence interval can now be obtained by picking the appropriate percentiles from this distribution.

Assumptions of the 95% Confidence Interval

The methods of computing 95% confidence intervals assume that the measurements taken from each person are independent of each other and that there are no systematic biases. These assumptions are subject to some criticism because measurement of nutrients is based not only on the amount of foods eaten, as given in the dietary survey, but also on food composition tables. The tables are themselves subject to variation, which is not taken into account in the estimate of the 95% confidence interval. The magnitude of this problem should be investigated through sensitivity analyses.

REFERENCES

Bickel, P. J., and K. A. Doksum. 1977. Mathematical Statistics: Basic Ideas and Selected Topics. Holden-Day, San Francisco.

Box, G. E. P., and D. R. Cox. 1964. An analysis of transformations. J. R. Stat. Soc. B 26:211-252.

Hoaglin, D. C., and F. Mosteller, eds. 1982. Understanding Robust and Exploratory Data Analysis. John Wiley & Sons, New York.

APPENDIX *D*

Algorithm for Computing the Probability of Intake Inadequacy

The probability approach described in this report depends on placement of the observed intake within a normalized distribution of requirements and calculation of the area under the normal distribution to the right of the observed intake. This is done by computing the Z value of the observed intake as:

$$Z = \frac{\text{Observed Intake} - \text{Mean Requirement}}{\text{Standard Deviation of Requirement}}.$$

The statistical tables of the standard normal distribution are then consulted to determine the area to the right of Z. This represents the probability that the intake is inadequate for the randomly selected person.

An algorithm for use on a computer gives very good agreement with published values of the area under the normal distribution (Abramowitz and Stegun, 1965). The following segment of a computer program illustrates the use of this algorithm. (The program segment is written in Applesoft Basic.)

```
1510   Z = (A(X) − NR)/(NR * CV)
1515   IF Z < 0 THEN Z = ABS(Z): VZ = 1
1520   IF Z > 10 THEN R = 0: GOTO 1545
1525   D1 = .0498673470: D2 = .0211410061: D3 = .0032776263:
       D4 = .0000380036: D5 = .0000488906: D6 = .0000053830
1530   G = 1 + D1 * Z + D2 * Z^2 + D3 * Z^3 + D4 * Z^4 + D5 * Z^5
       + D6 * Z^6
1535   R = 1/(2 * G^16)
1540   R = INT(R * 1000 + 0.5)/1000
1545   IF VZ < >0 THEN R = 1 − R: VZ = 0
1550   R(X) = R: R = 0
```

127

In this program, the following variables have been
generated before reaching the above program segment:
A(X) is the intake report for nutrient X; NR is the average requirement for nutrient X; and CV is the coefficient of variation of requirement for nutrient X,
expressed as a decimal rather than as a percentage. The
variables R and R(X) represent the calculated probability that the intake of nutrient X is inadequate to
meet the requirement for a person.

In the computations in this report, this algorithm
has been used with A(X) and R(X) representing the intakes
and risks for equal intervals of the population ranked by
level of intake (see Appendix A). The values of R(X)
have been summed across the population. This yields an
estimate of the prevalence of inadequate intakes within
the population, which is then divided by the population
size.

Computer routines are used to estimate requirements
on the basis of subject characteristics, to adjust requirement estimates for the additional needs of pregnancy or
lactation, and at the same time, to adjust variance estimates for the new requirement estimate. The program also
imputes weight or energy intake if not provided as input
(used in conjunction with derivation of a requirement
estimate for some nutrients) and again adjusts the variance of the derived requirement estimate to take into
account the variance associated with the imputed value.
This program was written for application to a particular
person. There are also algorithms for making equivalent
adjustments in the analysis of population data rather than
individual data if needed.

REFERENCE

Abramowitz, M., and I. A. Stegun, eds. 1965. Handbook
    of Mathematical Functions with Formulas, Graphs, and
    Mathematical Tables. Applied Mathematics Series No.
    55. National Bureau of Standards. U.S. Department of
    Commerce, Gaithersburg, Maryland.

Analysis of Error in the Estimation of Nutrient Intake Using Three Sample Data Sets

The impact of two different kinds of error on the prevalence estimate is described in Chapter 7. There, the subcommittee examined in detail two potential sources of error that can affect the estimation of nutrient intake:

- errors in estimating the composition of the food item consumed and

- errors in estimating or recording the amount of each food item consumed.

In this appendix, the committee examines the potential impact of unmeasured errors of this kind on the probability approach. A distinction will be made between random errors (deviations moving in both directions around a true mean) and systematic errors or biases (consistent under- or overestimation of the true value). A distinction will also be made between the impact of error in assessing a single serving of a single food and in calculating intake from a series of servings of foods in one day. Emphasis is placed on the effect of these errors on the estimated distribution of usual intakes across people rather than on actual intakes of particular individuals. These constructs are first illustrated using actual data, and then their theoretical implications are developed. The initial assumption of this analyses is that the food composition analyses are correct (e.g., no systematic bias) but that there is variation in reported composition.

VARIABILITY OF FOOD COMPOSITION

The most recent reference tables on food composition developed by the U.S. Department of Agriculture (USDA, 1976-1984) provide some information about the number of samples analyzed and the standard error of the mean for some foods. For these foods, the standard deviation (SD) of the nutrient composition can be calculated, and the coefficient of variation (CV = 100 x SD/mean) can be derived. Although the standard error (SE) is dependent upon the number of samples analyzed and describes the reliability of the estimate of the mean, the SD is not dependent on the number of samples per se (provided there are sufficient samples and analyses to supply a good description of the full range of foods) and furnishes a description of the range of values that can be taken by a specific sample of the food. The SE is a measure of the variability of the mean of the population and in that sense is a measure of the error that might be encountered in accepting the average composition of a particular food as the reference data. In the Chapter 6 analysis, therefore, the SE has been used to calculate confidence limits. For present purposes, however, the SD is more meaningful than the SE of the mean. The CV expresses this variability in relation to the mean, and it is useful in this exercise for comparing error in estimating nutrient content between several foods and for considering the impact of the error on the estimate of the daily intake of a nutrient, as used in dietary evaluation.

Because the SD cannot be estimated from the reference tables for all food items, the available SDs were examined and used to make a judgment about the possible CV or range of CVs that might apply for foods with missing data. The food composition tables indicate that the relative variability of micronutrients is greater than the variability of protein; this difference seems biologically plausible. The USDA provides no CV estimates for energy, because the reference data for energy concentration are computed rather than measured values.

Two kinds of data analyses were used to examine the impact of variability on dietary evaluation. In the first analysis, hypothetical variance estimates are assigned to a food record for a vegetarian diet. The variability estimates used for this analysis are shown in Table E-1. The subcommittee assumed that the magnitude of the CV is different for various nutrients, but the level of nutrient was not taken into account. Subsequent analyses, based as much as possible on

TABLE E-1.   Assumed Variability in Food Composition
Data Used in Estimating the Error[a]

Class of Vector	Range of CVs (%)
Energy	10-30
Protein	10-20
Other nutrients	10-45

[a]Data from G. H. Beaton, University of Toronto, personal communication, 1985.

reported variance estimates and complemented by imputed variances, are presented in a later section of this Appendix.

These variance estimates were applied with a simulation procedure to the dietary intake record of a vegetarian subject studied in Toronto. The food composition data reported by USDA (1976-1984) were used to estimate the average composition of each of the 21 foods included in the record. A variability was assigned to each food item by random selection within the ranges presented in Table E-1 by using the algorithm

$$CV \text{ (food item X)} = 10 + RND(1) \times Y,$$

where Y = 20 for energy, 10 for protein, and 35 for other nutrients. Thus, for each food item and each nutrient, there was a mean composition and CV. This procedure was used to randomly assign a specific composition for each food item or nutrient combination. A random value from the normal distribution, represented by the mean and CV for that food item, was chosen. Table E-2 presents the results that accrued from 1,000 repetitions of this exercise and computations of the SD and CV for the computed nutrient intake. The results show that the relative error is decreased for the total record of food intake in comparison to the individual food items. The exercise could be repeated by selecting new random values for the CVs of the food items and then obtaining composite error estimates, which would not be expected to differ markedly from those shown in Table E-2. The table also presents the direct calculation of the variances and the SD and CV of the total intake as the sum of variances of the individual item by conventional statistical approaches. Given the assumptions of normality for the individual composition distributions, this is a much more rapid approach than the

TABLE E-2.   Potential Error in a Person's Estimated
Nutrient Intake Attributable to Variance
in Food Composition Data on Sample
Vegetarian Diet[a,b]

Nutrient Vector	Food Composition Data						
	No Variance, Mean	With Variance Added to Food Compositions					
		By Randomization Approach			By Statististical Formula		
		Mean	SD	CV (%)	Mean	SD	CV (%)
Energy (kcal/day)	2,610.4	2,619.6	146.37	5.60	26,10.4	146.02	5.59
Protein (g/day)	68.8	68.7	3.96	5.76	68.8	4.04	5.87
Calcium (mg/day)	814.1	812.7	86.49	10.64	814.1	87.29	10.72
Iron (mg/day)	29.1	29.4	3.48	11.85	29.1	3.43	11.76
Vitamin A (IU/day)	13,085.5	13,070.0	1,912.67	14.63	13,085.5	1,880.3	14.37
Thiamin (mg/day)	2.3	2.3	0.3	12.69	2.3	0.29	12.73
Vitamin C (mg/day)	303.6	302.8	29.52	9.75	303.6	30.91	10.18

[a]Mean and standard deviations based on 1,000 iterations with normally randomized
variables in randomization approach. Statistical formula represents addition of
variances under the assumption that each variance is normally distributed with mean
and CV as described. For the CV of food composition randomly assigned to each
nutrient, see Table E-1. These CVs are as high as 45% for individual foods.
[b]Data from G. H. Beaton, University of Toronto, personal communication, 1985.

repeated calculations based on random selections. The comparison of the two methods in Table E-2 shows that the
results are practically identical.

A member of the subcommittee (H. Smiciklas-Wright, Pennsylvania State University, personal communication, 1985)
provided two food intake records for use in a second set of
analyses. New USDA food composition data and variance
estimates (reported standard errors and number of analyses) were available for most of the foods in these records
(USDA, 1976-1984). The data provided by Smiciklas-Wright
were used as more realistic examples for modeling the variance in estimated intake attributable to variability in the
food composition data.

The first step was to impute variabilities for food composition when they could not be derived directly from the
USDA tables. An internalized empirical exercise was used:
CVs were calculated for all foods, when data permitted, and
were plotted in relation to the level of nutrient reported

in the food. The plots suggested that the range of the CV
increased markedly at low concentrations of nutrient. This
increase may reflect limitations of methods for determining
food composition, because an absolute contribution of methodologic error may become a large relative error at the lowest
levels of nutrient concentration. Alternatively, it may
simply mean that at low levels, the biological variation is
not proportional to the mean. Nevertheless, it appears that
above a nutrient-specific break point, the variability seems
to relate to the mean, and the range of CVs is diminished.
This apparent relationship was used in imputing CVs in the
two sample diets in the exercise. The stratification of CV
ranges is shown in Table E-3.

Using the ranges shown in Table E-3 and the randomized
approach discussed earlier for the vegetarian diet, the subcommittee assigned estimates of variability to all foods for
which a direct derivation could not be made from data provided by the USDA. These data were then examined to determine the error in the estimated 1-day intake (see Table E-4).

TABLE E-3. Stratification of CV Ranges for Use in
Assigning Variability of Food Composi-
tion in Nonvegetarian Food Intake
Records[a]

Nutrient	Cutoff Point (per 100 g)	CV Range Assumed (%) Below Cutoff	Above Cutoff
Protein	2 g	5 - 50	5 - 15
Calcium	20 mg	5 - 50	5 - 15
Iron	1 mg	5 - 65	10 - 30
Magnesium	10 mg	5 - 50	10 - 30
Sodium	100 mg	5 - 65	5 - 15
Zinc	1 mg	5 - 65	10 - 30
Thiamin	0.05 mg	5 - 50	10 - 30
Riboflavin	0.05 mg	5 - 50	10 - 30
Niacin	0.5 mg	5 - 65	5 - 15
Vitamin C	7.5 mg	5 - 50	10 - 30
Vitamin B_6	0.1 mg	5 - 50	10 - 30
Folacin	20 mg	5 - 65	10 - 30
Vitamin A	300 IU	5 - 65	10 - 30

[a]Data from H. Smiciklas-Wright, Pennsylvania State
University, personal communication, 1985.

TABLE E-4. Comparison of Potential Error Due to Variability of Food Composition Associated with Estimated 1-Day Intakes, Non-vegetarian Diets[a,b]

| | Estimated 1-Day Intake | | | | | |
| | Diet HW1 | | | Diet HW2 | | |
Nutrient	Mean	SD	CV (%)	Mean	SD	CV (%)
Protein	104.6	6.20	5.93	97.5	2.21	2.27
Calcium	1,540.2	80.77	5.24	1,135.2	61.31	5.40
Iron	8.03	1.19	14.85	10.4	1.66	16.00
Magnesium	250.1	15.70	6.28	222.4	13.04	5.86
Sodium	4,129.5	157.36	3.81	2,589.8	121.73	4.70
Zinc	11.6	0.909	7.85	13.3	1.64	12.33
Thiamin	2.10	0.375	17.92	0.715	0.076	10.59
Riboflavin	2.60	0.205	7.90	2.13	0.154	7.22
Niacin	15.9	0.908	5.72	13.5	0.879	6.53
Vitamin B_6	1.45	0.136	9.37	1.43	0.210	14.62
Vitamin C	153.1	11.91	7.77	11.8	1.54	13.00
Folacin	184.3	19.80	10.74	97.1	12.02	12.38
Vitamin A	3,798.4	281.24	7.40	5,142.0	603.61	11.74

[a]Data from H. Smiciklas-Wright, Pennsylvania State University, personal communication, 1985.
[b]See Tables E-11 and E-12 for diet composition.

Here the variance of 1-day intake was computed by statistical algorithm rather than by simulation. For most of the foods reported in the first diet (HW1), there were standard errors from which variance estimates could be derived (see Tables E-9 through E-12 at the end of this appendix). The results are realistic estimates of the potential error of the estimated 1-day intake. For the second diet (HW2), a higher proportion of the variability for individual foods had to be imputed (see Table E-12).

Differences in the CV of the intake estimate for the two diets can be attributed to differences in variability associated with individual foods. The CV of the diet is also affected by the relative contributions to intake from individual foods with particularly high or low variabilities.

Effect of Increasing the Number of Foods in the Diet

Although it may not be apparent from a comparison of the three diets, it can be demonstrated by statistical theory that increasing the number of foods included in the record will decrease the relative variance of the total intake estimate. This effect is illustrated in Table E-5. In this model it is assumed that all foods make an equal contribution to total intake and thus exert the same impact upon variance of the sum. The table displays the impact of the number of foods in the record by using several hypothetical CVs for the food composition data.

RANDOM ERROR IN THE MEASUREMENT OF FOOD INTAKE

If the measurement or recording of actual intake of individual food items includes an implicit error because some items are underestimated and some are overestimated, then these measurements will lead to error in estimation of the 1-day intake of nutrients.

TABLE E-5.   Impact of the Number of Food Items in a Record on the Error Term for Computed Nutrient Intake[a]

Number of Foods in Record	CV (%) of Nutrient Content of Individual Food Serving				
	10	20	30	40	50
2	7.1	14.1	21.2	28.3	35.4
3	5.8	11.6	17.3	23.1	28.9
4	5.0	10.0	15.0	20.0	25.0
5	4.5	8.9	13.4	17.9	22.4
10	3.2	6.3	9.5	12.7	15.8
15	2.6	5.2	7.8	10.3	12.9
20	2.2	4.5	6.7	8.9	11.2
25	2.0	4.0	6.0	8.0	10.0
30	1.8	3.7	5.5	7.3	9.1

[a]These calculations assume that all foods make an equal contribution to the total intake and that all food servings have the same error terms. The values are based on a simulated distribution.

For analysis of measurement error when no variance in the food composition is taken into account, the considerations are identical to those discussed in the preceding section. The solution can be obtained by adding the variances, and the effects will be exactly as calculated for the variability of food composition tables.

When the model includes error both from measurement and from variation in food composition, the variance of a product must be computed. Statistical equations for the approximation of this variance have been developed by FAO/WHO/UNU (in press). If it is accepted that there is no correlation between the two variations, the following equation can be used to estimate the variance of the product of intake and food composition:

$$V = I^2 \times V_{(C)} + C^2 \times V_{(I)} + V_{(C)} \times V_{(I)},$$

where I^2 is the square of reported mean intake of units of food; C^2 is the square of reported mean concentration of nutrient per unit of food; V is the variance of content of a food whose content is I x C; $V_{(I)}$ is the variance of the intake measurement; and $V_{(C)}$ is the variance of the composition measurement. Thus the equation assumes no correlation between values of I and C, although approximations are available for situations in which there is a correlation. The result is a variance for each item that is then summed for the total intake.

To illustrate the impact of variation on estimations of the actual amount of the food items consumed, a hypothetical 10% CV for measurement will be assumed (see Table E-6). This illustration is based on the vegetarian diet described earlier. In the simulation, values were selected at random from two normal distributions (one for the intake estimate and one for the composition estimate) for each food item, and 1,000 iterations were performed. Using statistical calculations rather than the simulated approach, a member of the subcommittee performed a similar exercise for the data sets for diets HW1 and HW2.

Comparison of these variance estimates with those developed earlier for food composition alone reveal that the effect of adding a second source of variation, although real, is less than might have been anticipated. Unless the random error is very large, there will be a limited additional effect on the error term generated by food composition varia-

TABLE E-6. Error Term in 1-Day Intakes Associated with Variability
of Food Composition and Error in Intake Estimate in
Nonvegetarian Diets [a]

Nutrient	Diet HW1			Diet HW2		
	Mean	SD	CV (%)	Mean	SD	CV (%)
Protein	109.6	7.56	7.23	97.5	5.81	5.96
Calcium	1,540.2	103.7	6.74	1,135.2	82.52	7.26
Iron	8.03	1.23	15.35	10.40	1.73	16.62
Magnesium	250.0	17.72	7.08	222.4	15.51	6.97
Sodium	4,129.5	239.3	5.80	2,589.8	180.3	6.95
Zinc	11.58	1.00	8.67	13.32	1.76	13.22
Thiamin	2.10	0.395	18.85	0.716	0.080	11.13
Riboflavin	2.60	0.226	8.71	2.13	0.175	8.21
Niacin	15.89	1.18	7.43	13.46	1.29	9.49
Vitamin B_6	1.45	0.149	10.26	1.43	0.227	15.83
Vitamin C	153.1	14.78	9.65	11.85	1.61	13.56
Folacin	184.3	21.12	11.46	97.07	12.72	13.10
Vitamin A	3,798.4	313.2	8.25	5,142.0	683.0	13.28

[a]Data from H. Smiciklas-Wright, Pennsylvania State University,
personal communication, 1985. For composition of diets and food
composition variability estimates, see Tables E-11 and E-12. (CV
is based on the assumption that measurement error is 10% normally
distributed.)

bility. The estimates of protein intake in the HW1 data lead
to a 5.9% CV of the estimate of total protein intake when
only food composition variability is considered (see Table
E-7). However, when measurement error is added, the CV
increases to 7.2% (see Table E-6). For iron, the two CVs
are 14.9% and 15.4%.

The magnitude of the effect depends on many factors,
including the relative contributions of various food items
to the final intake (weighting of the relative variances);
the number of food items as discussed in the preceding section for food composition variation; and, importantly, the
magnitude of the two variances. Table E-8 illustrates the
effect of the estimated variability (error term) for an
individual food item when there is variability both in food
composition and in estimation of food quantity. As shown in
Table E-5, the relative variance of the total intake for many
individual foods would decrease as the number of foods
increases.

TABLE E-7. Error in 1-Day Intakes Attributable to Variability in Food Composition and Intake Estimate[a]

| Nutrient | Sample Diets | | | | | |
| | HW1 | | | HW2 | | |
	Mean	SD	CV (%)	Mean	SD	CV (%)
Protein	109.6	7.56	7.23	97.5	5.81	5.96
Calcium	1,540.2	103.7	6.74	1,135.2	82.52	7.26
Iron	8.03	1.23	15.35	10.40	1.73	16.62
Magnesium	250.0	17.72	7.08	222.4	15.51	6.97
Sodium	4,129.5	239.3	5.80	2,589.8	10.3	6.95

[a]Normally distributed with CV measurement error assumed to
be 10%.

TABLE E-8. Impact of Random Error in Intake and Food
Composition Data on the CV Calculated for
Nutrient Content of an Individual Serving
of Food[a,b]

| CV 2 | CV 1 | | | | |
	0	10	20	30	40
0	0	10	20	30	40
10	10	14.2	22.4	31.8	41.4
20	20	22.4	28.6	36.6	45.4
30	30	31.8	36.6	43.4	51.4
40	40	41.4	45.4	51.4	58.8

[a]Data from NFCS. Values are relative.
[b]All values expressed as CV = 100 x SD/mean. It is
not important to know which variable is 1 or 2. The
error term for a diet comprising several individual
servings of foods would necessitate a summation of
variances (see Table E-5).

These analyses demonstrate that the true intake of nutrients by a person on a particular day differs from the estimated intake and suggests that the standard deviation of this
error for mixed diets containing 15 to 20 different foods is
likely to fall in the range of 5% to 15%, depending on a
number of factors. Thus it can be assumed that 95% of the
time the estimated intake will fall within 10% to 30% of the
actual intake of a nutrient. The error in the estimate of a
particular person's intake on a certain day is appreciable.

CONCLUSIONS

These analyses demonstrate that random variation in food
composition (including random errors in analysis) and in the
estimation of food intake introduces an element of variation
in computed nutrient intake across days for 1-day records
and that the relative impact, although not as large as might
have been expected, is nevertheless real. These considerations suggest that part of the reported difference between
calculated intake and chemically determined intake for
duplicate meals or composite diets may arise from random
error and that perfect agreement should not be expected.

In considering the distributions of nutrient intake in
population data, the data on variability of food composition discussed in this appendix are not normally
included. That is, the true variability of 1-day intake is
greater than would be estimated with conventional techniques
based on average composition data from the food composition
table.

More important in the context of the present report is
the impact of random variation on estimation of the
prevalence of inadequate intake. Part of the unmeasured
variation associated with the 1-day intake estimate would
clearly be factored out by the analysis of variance (ANOVA)
procedure used to estimate the distributions of usual intake
in the population. This part of the variation would have no
final impact on the estimate of prevalence. Thus, there is
no need to measure or estimate its magnitude. To determine
if the entire effect is factored out in the ANOVA, a
statistical model was developed (see Chapter 8). For this
model, SEs were estimated from the food composition table
for the diet HW1 presented in this appendix.

A similar approach for deriving the SE of a 1-day intake was used to estimate the SD and CV, but SEs rather than SDs of composition of individual foods were used as the starting point. The results demonstrate that random variation as discussed in this appendix influences the confidence limits of the estimate of usual intake and may also influence the estimate of prevalence. If the prevalence estimate is below 50%, the effects will lead to a slight underestimation of the prevalence, and if the prevalence is above 50%, the effects will somewhat overestimate it. Fortunately, as demonstrated in Chapter 8, the under- or overestimations and the impact of confidence limits are not so great as to invalidate the approach to assessment. Nevertheless, it is clear that improvement of food composition data bases can improve the estimate of the prevalence of inadequate intake. True biological variation between individual samples of food will limit the improvement that can be gained. Modeling approaches such as those presented in this appendix together with those presented in Chapter 8 can be used to ascertain which types of improvements in the food composition data base would have the greatest impact on estimations of the prevalence of inadequate intakes. Analyses of this kind can provide the basis for establishing priorities for future analytical work.

True systematic biases in either food composition or food intake data are not considered in the analyses presented herein, but are discussed in Chapter 7. As was shown, these effects, if present, will influence the prevalence estimates. Elimination of systematic biases due to errors in methods should receive a high priority for this reason.

REFERENCES

FAO/WHO/UNU (Food and Agriculture Organization/World Health Organization/United Nations University). In press. Energy and Protein Requirements. Report of a Joint FAO/WHO/UNU meeting. World Health Organization, Geneva.

USDA (U.S. Department of Agriculture). 1976-1984. Composition of Foods: Raw, Processed, Prepared. Agriculture Handbook No. 8. Sections 1-12. Agricultural Research Service, U.S. Department of Agriculture, Washington, D.C.

TABLE E-9. Intake and Food Composition Data Used in the Computations Presented in Table E-2. CVs Assigned by Random Number Are Shown to the Right of Composition.[a]

Food Item	Weight Eaten (g)	Composition/100g												
		Energy		Protein		Calcium		Iron		Vitamin A		Thiamin		Vitamin C	
		kcal	%	g	%	mg	%	mg	%	IU	%	mg	%	mg	%
Watermelon	810	26	22	0.5	18	7	37	0.5	35	590	10	0.03	44	7	25
Cherries	515	70	22	1.3	14	22	32	0.4	24	110	38	0.05	21	10	22
Soy milk concentrate	125	126	12	4.8	16	30	27	0.8	33	0	--	0.06	19	0	--
Cereal mix	137	315	13	11.0	18	50	34	3.2	35	0	--	0.20	14	0	--
Figs	30	80	14	1.2	10	35	42	0.6	44	80	40	0.06	31	2	21
Lettuce	40	13	23	0.9	12	20	24	0.5	25	330	42	0.06	16	6	26
Cucumber	70	15	12	0.9	18	25	26	1.1	34	250	32	0.03	26	11	27
Tomato	80	22	15	1.1	17	13	39	0.5	22	206	43	0.06	30	20	40
Cabbage	110	24	10	1.3	10	49	21	0.4	37	130	43	0.05	13	47	37
Green peppers	15	22	18	1.2	15	9	10	0.7	20	420	17	0.08	12	128	25
Avocado	40	167	28	2.1	19	10	32	0.6	19	290	11	0.11	40	14	30
Olives	35	116	27	1.4	13	84	11	1.6	23	60	32	0	--	0	--
Green onions	15	45	28	1.1	16	51	31	1.0	23	2,000	44	0.05	30	32	42
Bread, white (nonmilk)	58	241	13	9.1	12	84	44	2.3	28	0	--	0.30	28	0	--
Mayonnaise	80	718	13	1.1	10	18	26	0.5	36	280	19	0.02	19	0	--
Corn on the cob	120	91	26	3.3	13	3	41	0.6	33	400	23	0.12	40	9	21
Peanut butter	32	580	19	25.2	16	395	21	2.0	20	0	--	0.12	21	0	--
Kidney beans	155	118	16	7.8	17	110	36	6.9	24	20	25	0.51	22	0	--
Celery	5	17	14	0.9	11	39	30	0.3	21	240	36	0.03	26	9	36
Cantaloupe	170	30	16	0.7	11	14	34	0.4	39	3,400	31	0.04	33	33	18
Black currants	10	54	23	1.7	15	60	15	1.1	22	230	22	0.05	15	200	44

[a]Based on a 1-day food intake record collected from a vegetarian. CV assigned by stratified random process. See text.

TABLE E-10. Example of the Application of Random Selection of Food Composition Estimates for Calcium[a]

Food Item	Tabulated Content (mg)	Hypothetical Calcium Content (mg in food consumed)									
		1	2	3	4	5	6	7	8	9	10
Watermelon	56	16	28	63	51	70	53	63	87	89	31
Cherries	113	185	178	184	134	90	67	191	190	140	77
Soy milk concentrate	38	40	46	53	52	16	37	42	32	52	25
Cereal mix	67	77	64	101	40	62	109	87	54	43	61
Figs	11	11	7	14	6	20	8	15	13	18	11
Lettuce	8	7	12	8	7	9	9	8	8	5	9
Cucumber	18	14	20	22	14	13	16	17	12	17	24
Tomato	10	2	13	12	6	14	10	19	13	15	9
Cabbage	54	75	48	40	62	35	51	74	64	57	44
Green peppers	1	1	1	2	2	1	1	1	1	1	1
Avocado	4	6	3	5	3	4	5	6	5	2	3
Olives	29	31	27	35	28	32	28	33	26	27	33
Green onions	8	8	9	8	5	5	11	9	7	10	8
Bread, white (nonmilk)	49	49	90	25	35	62	42	81	24	36	49
Mayonnaise	14	16	11	10	11	9	13	9	20	14	11
Corn on the cob	4	5	2	5	6	6	4	4	5	3	3
Peanut butter	126	134	143	136	131	142	102	148	166	157	104
Kidney beans	110	73	167	178	127	183	95	87	230	100	274
Celery	2	2	2	2	3	3	2	1	1	3	2
Cantaloupe	24	24	30	34	17	20	38	32	16	24	33
Black currants	6	6	8	6	6	4	5	6	7	8	7
Total	814	784	907	942	746	801	706	933	980	822	820

[a]Based on vegetarian diet described in Table E-9. Overall mean = 844.5; SD = 91.45; and CV = 10.83%.

TABLE E-11. Food Composition and Variability Estimates Associated with Nonvegetarian Food Record HW1[a]

Food Item	Weight Eaten (g)	Composition/100g											
		Protein		Calcium		Iron		Magnesium		Sodium		Zinc	
		g	%	mg	%	mg	%	mg	%	mg	%	mg	%
Orange juice	124	0.68	0.6	9	15.3	0.10	64.1	10	8.9	1	158.3	0.05	43.4
Scrambled egg	64	9.32	14.9*	74	13.1*	1.46	29.3*	12	21.4*	242	8.3*	1.10	28.1*
Sausage	26	13.80	13.4	--	--	1.13	15.4	12	18.8	805	7.5	1.87	14.3
Shredded wheat	28.4	11.00	3.5	38	15.8	4.22	12.7	132	15.0	10	93.0	3.30	14.0
Milk, whole	122	3.29	5.3	119	6.9	0.05	44.3	13	37.4	49	16.3	0.38	15.2
Coffee whitener	15	1.00	44.2	9	62.9	0.03	223.6	--	--	79	60.9	0.02	25.3*
Tomato soup	248	2.46	7.2*	64	14.6*	0.73	58.5*	9	11.8*	376	11.4*	0.117	27.5*
Frankfurters	90	11.28	5.2	11	2.0	1.15	29.3	10	9.8	1,120	8.4	1.84	14.0
Cheddar cheese	28	24.90	7.2	721	8.6	0.68	25.1	28	19.6	620	16.7	3.11	21.4
Peach	87	0.70	20.0	5	47.7	0.11	83.3	7	27.3	--	0	0.14	59.1
Milk shake	313	3.86	8.0	146	12.6	0.10	19.9	12	13.4	95	7.3	0.39	31.5
Potato soup	248	2.37	10.8*	67	14.8*	0.22	38.4*	7	34.2*	428	5.4*	0.072	55.0*
Pork chops	126	28.82	16.3	15	21.8*	0.81	16.7	30	23.7	67	6.3	2.38	14.6
Fruit cocktail	122	0.42	7.4	5	9.0	0.25	40.4	7	8.8	4	48.4	0.09	29.4*
Skim milk	245	3.41	4.3	123	13.3	0.04	38.2	11	17.0	52	27.1	0.40	36.9

Table continued on next page.

TABLE E-11. (Cont.)

Food item	Weight Eaten, (g)	Composition/100g Vitamin C mg	%	Thiamin mg	%	Riboflavin mg	%	Niacin mg	%	Vitamin B6 mg	%	Folate µg	%	Vitamin A IU	%
Orange juice	124	28.9	13.5	0.079	21.9	0.018	--	0.202	10.6	0.044	0	43.8	18.0	78.0	26.1
Scrambled egg	64	0.2	38.3*	0.061	18.3*	0.243	18.7*	0.066	52.0*	0.091	21.2*	35.0	28.0*	486.0	14.3*
Sausage	26	--	--	0.357	13.7	0.147	11.7	3.367	9.2	0.050	29.4	--	--	--	--
Shredded wheat	28.4	--	--	0.260	11.7	0.280	53.5	5.25	7.7	0.253	9.6	50.0	16.2	--	--
Milk, whole	122	0.94	50.2	0.038	27.6	0.162	14.0	0.084	15.7	0.042	49.4	5.0	28.3	126.0	34.5
Coffee whitener	15	--	--	--	--	--	--	--	--	--	--	--	--	89.0	82.9
Tomato soup	248	27.3	11.2*	0.054	12.6*	0.100	16.8*	0.613	12.9*	0.066	18.6*	8.4	37.1*	342.0	11.0*
Frankfurters	90	26	25.3	0.199	33.2	0.120	22.1	2.634	13.6	0.130	30.6	4.0	32.5	--	--
Cheddar cheese	28	--	--	0.027	55.0	0.375	24.9	0.080	67.6	0.070	46.2	18.0	55.8	1,059.0	25.2
Peach	87	6.6	37.8	0.017	35.3	0.041	19.5	0.990	4.4	0.018	23.6	3.4	28.2	535.0	10.2
Milk shake	313	--	--	0.030	33.9*	0.195	25.3*	0.146	22.0*	0.042	44.3*	7.0	56.1*	114.0	18.1*
Potato soup	248	0.5	16.1*	0.033	34.0*	0.095	21.0*	0.259	19.0*	0.036	14.7*	3.7	30.2*	179.0	36.6*
Pork chops	126	0.3	28.3	0.894	32.6	0.323	20.4	5.231	11.9	0.400	19.0	9.0	38.3*	6.0	6.2*
Fruit cocktail	122	2.1	33.6	0.016	19.8	0.011	--	0.363	21.9	0.052	29.9*	--	--	250.0	23.2
Skim milk	245	0.98		0.036		0.140		0.088		0.040		5.0		204.0	

aBased on dietary records (HW) provided by H. Smiciklas-Wright, Pennsylvania State University, personal communication, 1985. Number of items with imputed CV (*): protein, 3; calcium, 4; iron, 3; magnesium, 3; sodium, 3; zinc, 5; vitamin C, 8; thiamin, 7; riboflavin, 7; niacin, 7; vitamin B6, 10; folate, 7; and vitamin A, 9.

TABLE E-12. Food Composition and Variability Estimates Associated with Nonvegetarian Food Record HW2[a]

Food Item	Weight Eaten (g)	Composition/100 g											
		Protein		Calcium		Iron		Magnesium		Sodium		Zinc	
		g	%	mg	%	mg	%	mg	%	mg	%	mg	%
Grape juice	126	0.56	38.2	9	22.4	0.24	56.7	10	7.9	3	41.9	0.05	16.0
Farina, cooked	117	1.4	11.3*	2	45.3*	0.50	40.4*	2	15.4*	0	--	0.07	41.4*
Cream, half and half	121	2.96	5.8	105	9.2	0.07	25.7	10	13.5	41	7.1	0.51	49.2
Fried egg	46	11.7	5.7*	56	5.1*	2.01	23.7*	12	17.4*	312	11.8*	1.38	21.8*
Lemon juice	2.5	0.38	25.9	7	19.6	0.03	13.3	6	33.2	1	68.9	0.05	61.9*
Yogurt, low fat	227	5.25	10.9	183	11.7	0.08	20.0	17	11.8	70	38.5*	0.89	38.9
Vegetarian vegetable soup	241	0.87	13.2*	9	32.9*	0.45	58.4*	3	6.9*	341	8.7*	0.191	33.8*
Purple plums, canned	129	0.36	8.6	9	19.9	0.84	59.6	5	30.7*	19	29.0	0.07	37.9*
Whole chocolate milk	250	3.17	3.4	112	10.1	0.24	20.8*	13	10.7	60	19.4	0.41	12.0
Turkey, roast	170	29.5	2.2	20	15.5	1.96	22.0	26	1.6	67	8.6	3.04	4.1
Cranberry sauce	69	0.20	26.2*	4	37.2*	0.22	32.0*	3	30.5*	29	37.4*	0.05	63.7*
Green pea soup	250	3.44	12.1*	11	6.6*	0.78	57.6*	16	26.7*	395	5.9*	0.68	61.6*
Vanilla ice cream	133	3.61	15.8	132	11.7	0.09	49.5	14	9.3	87	29.3	1.06	62.4

Table continued on next page.

TABLE E-12 (Cont.)

Food Item	Weight Eaten (g)	Vitamin C mg	%	Thiamin mg	%	Riboflavin mg	%	Niacin mg	%	Vitamin B_6 mg	%	Folate μg	%	Vitamin A IU	%
Grape juice	126	0.10	36.4*	0.026	51.0	0.037	46.8	0.262	13.9	0.065	10.2	2.6	21.1	8	37.1*
Farina, cooked	117	0	--	0.08	27.5*	0.05	11.8*	0.55	5.9*	0.010	15.5*	2.0	12.0*	0	--
Cream, half and half	121	0.86	12.2*	0.035	30.0*	0.149	28.1*	0.078	38.4*	0.039	45.5*	2.0	26.0	434	15.6*
Fried egg	46	0	--	0.071	20.9*	0.257	12.3*	0.057	45.7*	0.109	17.1*	45.0	27.1*	622	10.6*
Lemon juice	2.5	45.0	20.4*	0.030	32.0*	0.010	23.8*	0.100	11.6*	0.051	11.6*	12.9	1.8	20	10.4*
Yogurt, low fat	227	0.80	70.7	0.044	19.7	0.214	13.2	0.117	50.0*	0.049	53.6*	11.0	23.6	66	27.7
Vegetarian vegetable soup	241	0.6	21.8*	0.022	47.3*	0.019	5.5*	0.380	54.9*	0.023	46.4*	4.4	9.5*	1,247	18.8*
Purple plums, canned	129	0.4	39.7	0.016	16.5	0.038	27.9	0.291	12.6	0.027	5.8*	2.5	65.0	259	59.1
Whole chocolate milk	250	0.91	27.6	0.037	46.2*	0.162	24.5*	0.125	49.2*	0.040	29.0*	5.0	62.6	121	27.9*
Turkey, roast	170	0	--	0.046	16.0	0.188	13.0	5.3	4.4	0.048	23.8*	8.0	24.2*	0	--
Cranberry sauce	69	2.0	14.5*	0.015	47.1	0.021	0	0.100	46.4	0.014	0	0	--	20	17.8*
Green pea soup	250	0.7	5.2*	0.043	35.4*	0.027	36.0*	0.496	44.9*	0.021	36.3*	0.7	43.5*	81	56.7*
Vanilla ice cream	133	0.53	45.9*	0.039	20.4	0.247	18.8	0.101	14.7	0.046	9.7*	2.0	19.2*	409	20.0

aNumber of items with imputed CV (*): protein, 5; calcium, 5; iron, 6; magnesium, 6; sodium, 5; zinc, 7; vitamin C, 8; thiamin, 7; riboflavin, 7; niacin, 7; vitamin B_6, 10; folate, 7; and vitamin A, 9.